Handbook of Esports Medicine

Lindsey Migliore • Caitlin McGee
Melita N. Moore
Editors

Handbook
of Esports Medicine

Clinical Aspects of Competitive
Video Gaming

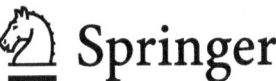 Springer

Editors
Lindsey Migliore
GamerDoc
Washington, DC
USA

Caitlin McGee
1HP
Washington, DC
USA

Melita N. Moore
Level Up Sports Medicine
Sacramento, CA
USA

ISBN 978-3-030-73609-5   ISBN 978-3-030-73610-1   (eBook)
https://doi.org/10.1007/978-3-030-73610-1

This Springer imprint is published by the registered company Springer Nature
Switzerland AG
The registered company address is: Gewerbestrasse 11, 6330 Cham, Switzerland

*Dedicated to Stella,
and bossy girls.*

Foreword

In my tenure as chief executive of Evil Geniuses, our grounding beliefs that gaming should be ubiquitous, and thus we offer a seat at the table for all the best esports athletes, go hand in hand with physical and mental wellness.

Also, in my tenure in esports, it never failed to surprise me how that idea, when broached with others in the space, received a response as if it were iconoclastic and novel. But health and wellness for athletes, even player athletes, is not a radical idea. When you devote your entire livelihood to a dream and a demanding activity, you must be holistically prepared and supported to execute at the highest level. However, until now, our player athletes have been failed by the industry and infrastructure, as the support around the legitimacy of holistic wellness, was insufficient and non-existent.

When I was approached by Dr. Migliore about the creation of an esports medicine handbook, I could only feel relief – like a large weight had been lifted from my back. But let me clarify – relief not because of pride of inclusion, or of the opportunity to showcase my (mediocre) writing skills, but relief in the fact that tenured, brilliant, and passionate medical professionals had taken the time and diligence to tirelessly collaborate, think through, and put forth a much-overdue source of knowledge on esports health and medicine.

When developing competitive esports champions, I remember entering the space a few years ago to find myself bewildered at the lack of robust and holistic support for these player athletes. I use "athlete" on purpose – mental, physical, and emotional health are all necessary for top tier competitive play. Yet it was an under-served and underdeveloped sector of the competitive ecosystem.

But this is ludicrous, as player churn is high due to injury at a relatively young age compared to traditional sports – eye strain, carpal tunnel, psychological lack of support, the list goes on – we all do ourselves a disservice to the development of the esports space. We also do ourselves a horrendous disservice to the *humans* who have put their all into their sport and have sacrificed their future to excel today.

While most people know myself as the esports CEO that her-alded from private equity, what most people do not see is the esports CEO that fell in love with non-traditional competitive sports since my teen years. In an earlier life, I coached Tae Kwon Do. I lived and breathed the importance of instilling mental and physical wellness – and toughness – into those as young as four. I lived the reality of how one's sport can be their escape, their opportunity, their life. I see esports as no different – and the focus, seriousness, and passion carry through. Martial arts created me, and the focus on mental and physical coaching was paramount throughout my life.

This focus carries over to me as a team owner, as I want the best players to compete at their fullest, and when they leave my team – as they all must one day – they leave as healthy and ethical humans, prepared for what comes next.

My player athletes are not assets to me, for lifting trophies, or building brands. They are unique and diverse human beings, who have trusted me to help them develop, grow, and fulfill their ambi-tions. They come from all walks of life, all genders, all sexual orientations, all creeds, and for me to be nimble in their holistic support is an absolute must. But I am not a medical expert, and the resources for me to do this did not exist.

This is known by your wonderful authors, a diverse, intelli-gent, and progressive group of doctors, physical therapists, per-sonal trainers, and researchers, who deeply know the interconnectedness of the human body, mind, and output. Their sacrifice and focus to provide a guiding text that will create a sturdy foundation for the prosperity of the esports industry and their athletes should matter to more than just team owners.

Fans should rejoice that their beloved players and personalities are getting the support they need to live a full and safe career. Industry professionals and the competitive ecosystem should celebrate as the mass-acceptance of the legitimacy and importance of esports and its athletes expands. And for the curious mind, rejoice that you get to observe progress being made in the future of a global sustainable entertainment and sport.

Physical and mental health cannot be overlooked, and I am grateful to have the opportunity to introduce you to a lynchpin and industry-revolutionizing text.

Nicole LaPointe Jameson
Evil Geniuses
Seattle, WA, USA

Preface

Esports medicine is a field in its infancy. Competitive gaming has exponentially grown in the past years, with revenues reaching billions. Athletes, motivated by the idea of playing video games for a real salary, "grind" for excessive hours to turn their dream into reality. Without adequate support or informed healthcare professionals, most are forced into retirement just after reaching their twenties.

This book serves as an introduction to the field of esports, as well as to the specific injuries and disorders that affect patients with this unique lifestyle. Practitioners will not only be educated what exactly competitive gaming truly is but also each ailment that corresponds to the playstyle.

As with any origin story, the field of esports medicine still has an incredible future ahead of it, and much to learn. Current data and recommendations are based on case and observational studies, or extrapolated from similar populations. Those who wish to pursue this path must do so with an open, inquisitive, and creative mind, as well as an understanding that this is a field unlike any other.

Washington, DC, USA   Lindsey Migliore
Washington, DC, USA   Caitlin McGee
Sacremento, CA, USA   Melita N. Moore

Acknowledgments

This would not have been possible without the tireless support of our friends and families. It was written well past office hours, late into the night, and during a pandemic. Thank you to Amber for the never-ending encouragement and limitless patience, Marken for always making things look beautiful, and Sarah for bringing this over the finish line. Thank you to Craig for your confidence, reassurance, and spreadsheets.

Thank you to our amazing contributing authors for their hard work, independence, and commitment to excellence.

To the team at Springer, specifically Kristopher Spring and Richard Lansing, thank you for your courage to be the first. We're thrilled to be able to share our knowledge, experience, and passion with all who want to learn.

Contents

About the Editors

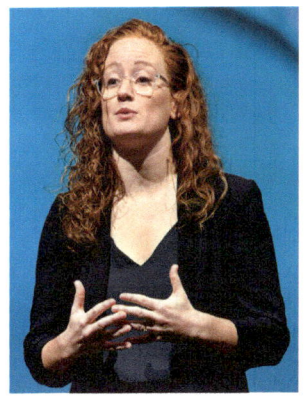

Lindsey Migliore is a board certified physician in the field of physical medicine and rehabilitation. She has dedicated her career to advancing the field of esports medicine and creating a healthier, more equitable gaming industry. She is the founder of GamerDoc, the executive director of Queer Women of Esports, a faculty associate for the NYIT Center for Sports Medicine, and an editor for the Annals of Esports Research. She is a proud graduate of Wellesley College.

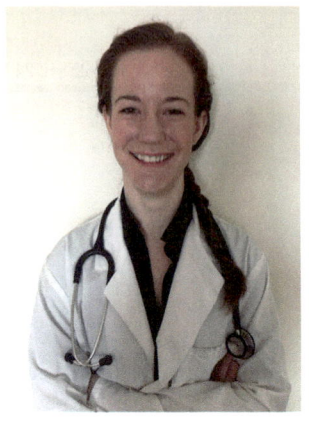

Caitlin McGee, PT, DPT, MS received her undergraduate degree in neuroscience and exercise and sport science from Ursinus College and her doctorate in physical therapy from the University of Delaware. She has been working in esports and orthopedic medicine for 6 years. She is the co-owner and performance and esports medicine director of 1HP, a company that provides health and performance services to players, teams, and school esports programs, as well as a co-founder of the Esports Health and Performance Institute. Her areas of interest include the effects of exercise on player performance, player perceptions of pain, and the impact of mental health on pain and physical function in gamers.

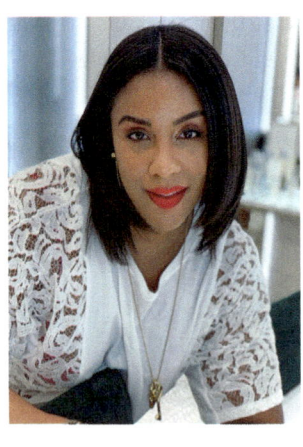

Melita N. Moore is a quadruple board certified physician in physical medicine and rehabilitation, sports medicine, brain injury medicine, and lifestyle medicine at MedStar Health System in Washington, DC. She serves as a team physician in the NBA 2K League, WNBA, and NBA G League. She is one of a few team physicians of a professional esports team in the USA and is an international leader on health and wellness for gamers. In addition, she is a member of the board and chair of the Health and Wellness

Commission for the Global Esports Federation. Her goal is to educate parents, gamers, and stakeholders on the importance of healthy lifestyles in a digital world.

List of Contributors

Kristen Beckman, MS, OTR/L Upper Marlboro, MD, USA

Carl Daubert, MS Performance Coach Carl Consulting, Hanover Township, PA, USA

Christopher Ferguson, PhD Department of Psychology, Stetson University, DeLand, FL, USA

Rachel Kowert, PhD TakeThis, Seattle, WA, USA

Lauren Trocchio, MSc, RD, CSSD, CSOWM, LD Nutrition Unlocked, LLC, Arlington, VA, USA

What Is Esports? The Past, Present, and Future of Competitive Gaming

Lindsey Migliore

1.1 Introduction

In 1958, hundreds of students lined up for an analog computer at the Brookhaven National Laboratory. Over the next three days, thousands would play the world's first-ever game designed for entertainment purposes only, Tennis for Two.

Since then, video games have exponentially evolved from their basement laboratory ancestral roots. Competitions, originally begun as a friendly split-screen match between friends or a quest for an arcade high score, have followed a similar growth trajectory. Competitive video gaming, known as esports, has exploded in popularity in recent years. With over 450 million viewers worldwide and almost $1 billion in revenue in 2020, esports is not a fad, but rather a technological and cultural phenomenon [1].

> **Esports Versus eSports**
> The stylization of esports has come under debate in recent years. In 2017, the Associated Press (AP) settled on "esports" over "eSports" or "e-sports." Some organizations named prior to 2017 have chosen to retain their original stylization, but the authors recommend utilizing the AP stylization.

L. Migliore (✉)
GamerDoc, Washington, DC, USA
e-mail: doc@gamerdoc.net

© The Author(s), under exclusive license to Springer Nature Switzerland AG 2021
L. Migliore et al. (eds.), *Handbook of Esports Medicine*,
https://doi.org/10.1007/978-3-030-73610-1_1

To remain competitive in this popular and sometimes lucrative field, gamers often practice upwards of 12 hours a day, performing anywhere from 400–600 actions per minute. As such, they are susceptible to a unique set of injuries and disorders from these complex movements, extended screen time, and sedentary tendencies. This population needs motivated and educated healthcare providers familiar with their lifestyle and ailments to effectively prevent, diagnose, and treat relevant esports medical conditions.

This chapter will impart the fundamental basics of esports necessary to understand the terminology and culture of competitive video gaming.

1.2   History

Almost 50 years prior to when over 100 million viewers tuned in for the League of Legends World Championships, the first esports tournament was held. 24 players competed in a Spacewar tournament at Stanford University on October 19, 1972. The 2019 champions were rewarded with $834,000 and a trophy designed by Louis Vuitton. The 1972 winners received an annual subscription to Rolling Stone magazine.

The evolution of esports has always been closely tied to technological advancements. Before powerful computers were made affordable and lightning fast internet was seen as a right rather than a privilege, arcades and the eternal quest for a high score (Fig. 1.1) became the epicenter of early esports. A three-letter abbreviation, traditionally meant to display a player's initials but used more creatively by some, displayed publicly and proudly for all other players to gaze upon, catalyzed the competition. In 1983, the United States National Video Game Team (USNVGT) was formed, laying the groundwork for esports organizations of modern day.

In the 1990s, personal computers (PCs) and consoles became more reasonably priced, and subsequently more commonplace. The evolution of the internet allowed multiple computers to be simultaneously connected, enabling more complex multiplayer

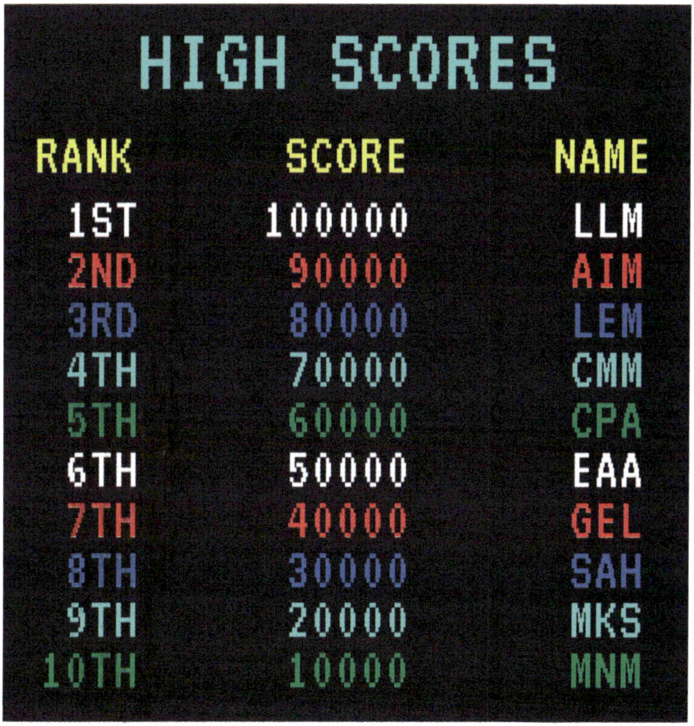

Fig. 1.1 Arcade high scores, depicted in brightly colored letters, served as the earliest origins of competitive gaming. Three-letter abbreviations typically signified a player's initials, and corresponded to the highest point total in the game

engagements. In the mid-1990s, local area network (LAN) parties emerged. The concept of a LAN party is simple. Bring your own PC or console, connect them together, and compete for prizes ranging anywhere from bragging rights to large sums of cash [2].

As technology continued to mature, computers with greater processing power allowed for more advanced games to be developed. However, for the average person they still lacked general affordability. The Internet cafe served as a compromise. Gamers could rent time on PCs to engage in multiplayer games for a low hourly rate.

While participation in gaming became more accessible, viewership still required physical attendance and subsequently lagged behind. This changed in the early 2010s with the availability of online streaming services, allowing tournaments to be broadcasted for anyone with an internet connection to view.

In the late 2010s, esports became more mainstream as popular gaming titles formed competitive leagues and tournaments vastly expanded. With this expansion came a vibrant culture shift. In the public eye, the gamer was being seen less as a basement-dwelling sluggard and more as a talent, leading to the beginnings of acceptance of the "pro-gamer" as a viable career path.

The education system served an integral role in organizing video game play. While high school and college gaming clubs have been in existence for decades, varsity esports teams at the collegiate level were relatively unheard of prior to the late 2010s. College organizations, with similar levels of institutional support as the traditional athletics teams, began competing in regional brackets. In 2018, Harrisburg University awarded full-ride scholarships to its entire esports roster, becoming the first institution to do so.

Dedicated spaces for esports also began to flourish around the same time frame. In 2015, the Esports Arena opened in Santa Ana, California, and multiple indoor arenas dedicated to hosting esports events followed suit. In 2019, during the Eighth Olympic Summit, the International Olympic Committee announced it would consider sports-simulation games for an official Olympic event in the distant future.

At the close of the 2010s, esports viewership in the United States had already eclipsed that of any other professional sport aside from football. Total tournament earnings for 2019 was a quarter of a billion dollars. The rich history of competitive video gaming is set to eclipse records and gain further popularity in the 2020s.

1.3   Console Versus Computer Gaming

Game titles are played primarily on a personal computer or console. The mechanics of play differs drastically, depending on choice, and dictate injury susceptibilities. An understanding of the input devices is essential for any healthcare provider wishing to provide care to esports athletes.

1.3.1   Console Gaming

A video game console is used to describe a computer designed primarily for game playing. Current popular brands include the Microsoft Xbox, Sony Playstation, and Nintendo Switch.

Players employ hand-held controllers as the primary input device for movements and actions. The typical anatomy of a controller is shown in Fig. 1.2. While the design varies between brands, the dual analog stick has become the most popular configuration. Two analog sticks are arranged on opposite sides, each to be controlled by either thumb. The analog sticks function primarily in movement control (similar to a computer mouse), and have largely replaced the traditional gamepad. Specialized variants exist for specific games, such as steering wheels for driving games, or arcade sticks for fighting games.

The controller also features buttons, triggers, or paddles on one or more sides. The physical mechanism by which players reach the buttons tends to vary based on preference and title being played, and will be discussed in depth in Chap. 5.

Claw Grip

"The claw" is an alternative grip used to reach the buttons on the front side of the control, while keeping the thumbs on the analog stick. The index finger is abducted and maximally flexed at the proximal and distal interphalangeal joint.

DIRECTIONAL BUTTONS   **BILATERAL TRIGGERS**   **ACTION BUTTONS**

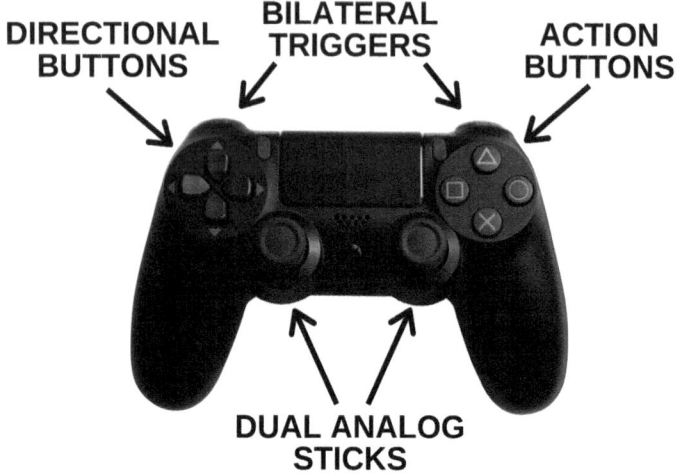

DUAL ANALOG STICKS

Fig. 1.2 The anatomy of a controller. Directional buttons, also known as a "D-pad" are on the left side. Originally, but still occasionally used for movement until the popularity of the analog sticks, they often correspond to less-commonly used actions. Two pairs of triggers top the cranial section of the controller. Action buttons, either designated by shapes, letters or numbers frame the right side. Dual analog sticks, the hallmark of the modern design, sit either directly across from one another, or staggered, depending on the brand

1.3.2 Computer Gaming

1.3.2.1 Personal Computer (PC) Gaming, Mouse and Keyboard Gaming

While a home computer is often utilized for casual PC gaming, more serious competitors have specialized "builds" with exponentially more robust computing power. The input devices are most commonly a computer keyboard and mouse.

Specialized gaming mice are available with lightweight designs and additional buttons on the sides. The mouse is generally held with three different grips, and the specific ergonomics of each are discussed in detail in Chap. 5.

1. Palm: The palm is in contact with the proximal mouse, and fingerpads are in full contact with the distal mouse.
2. Claw: Metacarpophalangeal flexion coupled with wrist extension places less of the palm in contact with the mouse, and only the distal phalanges. This allows for more precise movements.
3. Tip: The palm is completely lifted from the mouse, with only the distal tips of the fingers being used to control movement.

The keyboard can be used in a variety of fashions. For games involving avatar control, the classic "WASD" keyboard is used for movement with the left hand, with the ring finger on A (move left), middle switching between S (move back) and W (move forward), and index on D (move right). Thus, the term "W Key" denotes an aggressive, forward dominated play style as a player's finger does not leave the "move forward" button.

When gaming, keyboards are frequently angled differently from a traditional horizontal position, as shown in Fig. 1.3. This practice was started in Internet cafes, where narrow desks limited the range of mouse movement. In lieu of sacrificing accuracy, keyboards are turned completely vertical, allowing for wider mouse territory. Vertical keyboards are still in usage outside of Internet cafes for reasons ranging from personal preference, ease of handling, and faster actions.

1.4   Esports Genres

The breadth of video game titles available for play rivals that of any other form of entertainment. While competitive play exists for everything from casual mobile games to farming simulators, titles are often separated by "tiers." Originally developed by Jen Hilgers, games are placed into one of three tiers based on prize pool amounts, hours watched, and social media impact. While the topic is in itself largely controversial due to personal opinions and debates on method of calculation, the following genres are generally considered tier-level esports [3].

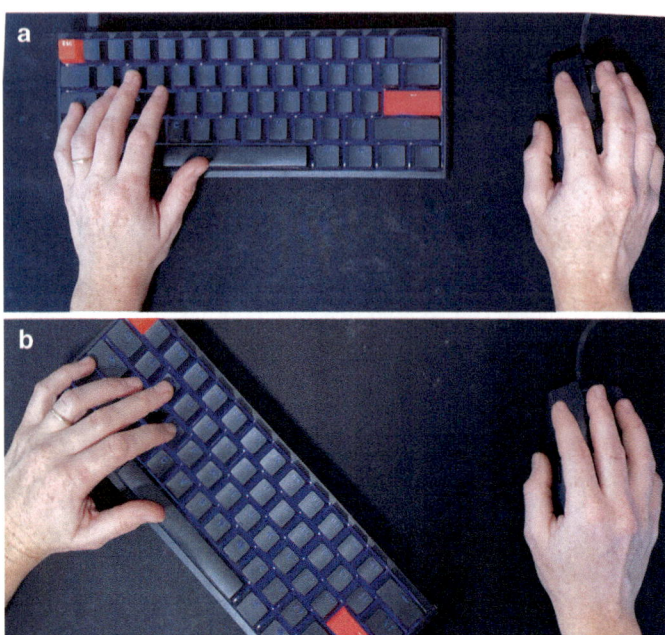

Fig. 1.3 Horizontal versus vertical keyboard orientations. (**a**) The traditional horizontal orientation employed by non-gamers and the casual gaming population. The player's left hand rests on the keyboard, typically on the WASD keys for first- and third-person games, and the right hand utilizes the mouse for aiming and targeting purposes. (**b**) The vertical orientation involves turning the keyboard somewhere between 0 to 90°, freeing up more space for mouse movement

1.4.1 First-Person Shooter

1.4.1.1 Call of Duty, Overwatch, Counter-Strike: Global Offensive, Halo, Rainbow 6 Siege

First-person shooter (FPS) is a genre centered around weapons-based combat through the eyes of the game's character (first-person view). This is in contrast to third-person games, where players can see the body of the character they control.

Across titles, similar game modes are utilized. The most traditional game mode is "Deathmatch", where points are awarded for enemy eliminations. The "Kill to Death", or "K:D" ratio is the amount of enemy kills versus the times a player themselves died, with a higher number signifying greater success.

Other popular game modes include video game versions of capture the flag and queen of the hill, where players must hold onto a landmark for a period of time, with that landmark often switching after a set period. Respawning, that is, returning to life after being eliminated by the opposing team is common. Players generally respawn in areas near where their teammates are located.

Spawn Camping

Spawn camping is the practice of positioning oneself in direct sight of the opposing team's spawn location, with the goal of immediately eliminating them upon respawning, and subsequently having no chance of defense.

FPS games are typically one of the most popular genres in the casual gaming population. Although there is limited data on esports, evidence suggests that playing FPS games promoted greater cognitive flexibility, as demonstrated by greater performance on a task-switching paradigm [4].

1.4.2   Battle Royale

1.4.2.1 PlayerUnknown's Battlegrounds (PUBG), Fortnite, Apex Legends, H1Z1, Call of Duty: Warzone

The Battle Royale genre (BR) blends classic elements of survivalism with last-person standing. Either first- or third-person point of views are applied. The overarching goal is to scavenge for supplies while avoiding being eliminated by enemies. Games often employ the same mechanics, with players randomly spawned or dropped onto a map from an aircraft. The maps are often identical game-to-game, with weapons, equipment, and consumables varying locations each time based on a random number generator (RNG). Players will have no or only basic weapons in the beginning, and may acquire and upgrade their items during the course of the match. As enemies are eliminated, the "safe area" of the map shrinks, drawing survivors towards the center. Once eliminated, players often do not respawn and must start another match. The winner is the last player or team alive [5].

> **Origin Story**
> One of the original BR games, PlayerUnknown's Battlegrounds, was based on the 2000 Japanese film "Battle Royale".

1.4.3   Real-Time Strategy

1.4.3.1 Starcraft, Warcraft

Strategy video games are often based on planning and tactical decision making to achieve victory. The category is subdivided based on whether play proceeds in a turn-based or real-time fashion. Real-time strategy (RTS) games are by far the most popular in esports.

In typical RTS titles, players are given a bird's eye view of the map, over which resources are splayed. The player operates in a god-like capacity, often controlling multiple avatars at once. Victory is achieved by completing certain objectives while utilizing common themes: resource management, base construction, and technological advancement. Resources can be gathered from the environment, which are used to create units and structures. There is often a technological side to the game as well, with more advanced upgrades conveying a tactical advantage.

Both micro- and macromanagement skills are needed. Each individual unit constantly requires specific instruction, yet the overall objective must be simultaneously worked towards, often to build a large and more skillful army than the opponent.

This subgenre is most commonly played on PC, with the mouse used to navigate the map and select units or targets. The "Click and Drag" technique is applied by clicking a space and dragging the mouse over multiple units. Keyboard buttons coincide with different commands, and actions per minute (APMs) in RTS games can exceed 600.

1.4.4   Multiplayer Online Battle Arena

1.4.4.1 Defense of the Ancients (Dota), League of Legends (LoL), Smite

Originally classified as a subgenre of strategy games known as "action real-time strategy" (ARTS), multiplayer online battle arena (MOBA) titles have earned their own category. As opposed to directing multiple units and avatars at once, the integral difference between RTS and MOBA is that only one main avatar is controlled, often called "heroes." Furthermore, players may work cooperatively with other teammates, usually in squads of five, towards common objectives. Non-player characters (NPCs) spawn on the map, offering each player an advantage or additional obstacle.

Maps often utilize isometric graphics, a viewpoint that is a cross between top-down and side view, effectively producing a three-dimensional effect and allowing the environment to be visualized from an entirely different angle than other genres.

Victory is often achieved either via eliminating every member of the opposing team, or by destroying the enemy's main structure. These structures are reached by progressing down predetermined paths in the map, often called lanes. Throughout these lanes are other structures that may spawn NPCs or deal damage, which can be captured and controlled. Players may also be designated by which lane they attack down, as a "Top Lane" "Mid Lane" or "Bottom Lane."

Team Composition
Heroes have varying abilities and skills that are designed to complement other team members. The common classes are "tank," "healer," and "damage-per-second," Tank classes are designed to draw the enemies' attention while taking large amounts of damage. Healer, or other support classes, keep teammates alive and may offer other unique support skills. Damage-per-second (DPS) characters are designed to reign damage. Overwatch, a popular FPS title, relies heavily on team composition.

1.4.5   Fighting

1.4.5.1 Street Fighter (SFV), Tekken, Mortal Kombat, Dragon Ball FighterZ, Injustice, Skullgirls

Player-controlled characters battle each other in a fixed-space, close-quarters environment. Traditionally, all players share the same sideways, 2D viewpoint. The primary objective is to deplete your opponent's health bar to zero over multiple rounds (typically a best of three format).

Players can choose from a multitude of characters, each with their own distinct attacks, counterattacks, and blocks. Each character has their own set of moves, with more complex combinations corresponding to more powerful attacks (special attacks). Unlike FPS, RTS, and MOBA genres, fighting games are more commonly played on consoles with portable arcade sticks or controllers. While traditional titles like Tekken and Mortal Combat are one-versus-one, Super Smash Bro allows for more than two characters to battle at one time.

> **FGC**
> The fighting game community is often abbreviated as FGC.

1.4.6   Digital Collectible Card Game

1.4.6.1 Hearthstone

The popularity of digital collectible card games (DCCGs) was heralded by that of collectible card games like Magic the Gathering and Pokemon, and borrow the same mechanics. They can also be classified as turn-based strategy games.

Players manage a personalized collection of cards that they do battle against an opponent with, typically in a one-versus-one format. Cards may signify the introduction of a character, a spell, or power up. The goal is to use the deck to reduce an opponent's health to zero. More powerful cards can be obtained via gameplay, which are in turn used to build more powerful decks.

1.4.7   Sports Simulation

1.4.7.1 NBA2K, NHL, Rocket League, FIFA

Simulation games are intended to closely copy real-world activities, most commonly a sport. Sports simulation games are often named after the traditional athletics organization they emulate. Unlike other genres, where years or decades may go by before a new title is released, updated sports simulation games are often released annually.

Players control characters that usually represent real athletes, with statistics modeled after their actual height, weight, and skill sets. The notable exception to these concepts is Rocket League, which has been appropriately described as "flying car soccer." Players guide cars inside of a giant arena with the overall goal of knocking a giant ball into your opponent's net.

1.5   Competitions

Organized esports play can take a variety of forms, with leagues and tournaments among the most common.

In league play, professional teams field elite lineups to compete against other professional teams throughout a season. Teams may be promoted or relegated to lower leagues, depending on their performance throughout the year.

More recently, competitive dynamics have shifted towards the traditional sports franchise model as esports finds more mainstream success and higher viewership. By removing the relegation and promotion dynamics, teams operate on a more permanent and thus more reliable basis. This fosters stable fan bases, and larger and more consistent investments.

In 2017, Riot Games and Blizzard Entertainment began operations of the North American League of Legends Championship Series and the Overwatch League (OWL). The OWL was formed from 12 international teams. These teams competed throughout a season, each vying for a finite number of playoff spots. Playoffs culminated in a championship match which crowned one team supreme. Since then, the NBA2K League (basketball), eMLS (soccer), and Call of Duty League have all followed suit. Franchise teams often pay their players a salary, rather than relying on prize money for compensation [6].

Tournaments continue to remain popular in non-team-based titles. Individuals or squads participate in qualifiers, which may be open to the public or by invitation only. This initial stage may be remote, with matches played online. While this favors the non-professional player who may not have the time or resources to engage in competitive gameplay outside of their home, it allows for an element of cheating or hacking as there are obviously no referees present. Once qualified, most tournaments involve physical travel and competition on a group stage.

Local area network (LAN) tournaments were arguably the birthplace of esports, and are still popular amongst amateur video gamers. Tournaments are held in venues ranging from basements to convention centers.

The tournament model favors amateur players, as they do not have to be drafted or recruited to a specific team to compete. Prize money for tournaments can range from meager to millions of dollars. In July 2019, the Fortnite World Cup awarded $30 million in prize money in a single weekend.

1.6   Video Game Live Streaming

While competition is what inherently defines esports, video game live streaming, known simply as "streaming" for short, offers an alternative way to earn income. Gameplay is broadcasted live, though websites such as Twitch, Mixer (Microsoft's streaming service that shutdown in 2020), YouTube Gaming, and Facebook Gaming. Popular streamers such as Ninja and Shroud often broadcast for up to 100,000 viewers at one time, and can earn incomes that exceed several million dollars a year [7].

With streaming, entertainment rather than competition is rewarded. Subsequently, this favors more unique and captivating personalities rather than the best and most talented player.

1.7   Conclusion

Esports earnings in 2021 are expected to exceed one billion for the very first time, marking a gigantic milestone. If viewership trends continue at the current trajectory, these numbers will only continue to grow. Despite the explosion of esports participants, leagues, tournaments, and sponsors, stigma and naivety still impedes the professional gamer from being seen as any other person whose success and career depends on the performance of their body and mind: an athlete.

Remaining competitive in this field requires the same amount of physical and mental training and commitment as any other form of professional athletics. Instead of running sprints and lifting weights, esports athletes are cementing complex motor patterns involving miniscule muscles of the hand and perfecting their hand eye coordination. In lieu of a gym, gamers prepare in a cooled and darkened room, often lit only by the glow of a computer monitor and LED lights of a specialized gaming PC.

Gamers are susceptible to their own unique set of injuries and illness that necessitates the attention of healthcare providers knowledgeable of their lifestyles, training schedules, and play mechanics.

References

1. Newzoo. Global esports market report. 2019. https://resources.newzoo. com/hubfs/2019_Free_Global_Esports_Market_Report.pdf?utm_ campaign=Esports%20Market%20Report. Accessed 7 Jan 2020.
2. Kent S. The ultimate history of video games. New York: Random House International; 2002.
3. Hilgers J. Esports games tiers. 2017. https://esportsobserver.com/esports-games-tiers. Accessed 7 Jan 2020.
4. Colzato LS, van Leeuwen PJ, van den Wildenberg WP, Hommel B. DOOM'd to switch: superior cognitive flexibility in players of first person shooter games. Front Psychol. 2010;1:8. https://doi.org/10.3389/fpsyg.2010.00008.
5. Fillari A. Battle royale games explained: Fortnite, PUBG, and what could be the next big hit. 2019. https://www.gamespot.com/articles/battle-

royale-games-explained-fortnite-pubg-and-wh/1100-6459225/. Accessed
7 Jan 2020.
6. Seiner J. What's overwatch? Why is it on ESPN? 8 things to know about
competitive gaming. 2018. https://www.chicagotribune.com/sports/
breaking/ct-spt-overwatch-league-esports-espn-20180726-story.html.
Accessed 7 Jan 2020.
7. Chaloner P, Sillis B. This is esports (and how to spell it). London: Blooms-
bury Sport; 2020.

Upper Extremity Disorders in Esports

2

Lindsey Migliore and Kristen Beckman

2.1 General

Arguably, the most important and essential parts of a gamer's body are their hands. Observational data has found that actions per minute for games like Starcraft II can reach upwards of 300–600. That breaks down to 10 actions per second. With a total of 34 individual muscles coordinating those delicate movements, a multitude of issues can arise.

Injuries to the upper extremity in the esports population most likely result from chronic microtraumas rather than acute processes. As a result, symptoms may be insidious, and worsen slowly, often below the threshold of a player's consciousness.

Furthermore, because of the high level of importance placed on the upper extremity, exploration of how the symptoms have affected the player's functionality is critically important. What are they prevented from doing because of the symptoms? If the answer is nothing, then focus should be placed on prevention and

L. Migliore (✉)
GamerDoc, Washington, DC, USA
e-mail: doc@gamerdoc.net

K. Beckman
Upper Marlboro, MD, USA

© The Author(s), under exclusive license to Springer Nature Switzerland AG 2021
L. Migliore et al. (eds.), *Handbook of Esports Medicine*,
https://doi.org/10.1007/978-3-030-73610-1_2

17

rehabilitation. If players have begun to adjust their play style or lifestyle as a result, such as switching keybinds due to discomfort or weakness, then more aggressive treatment is warranted. As with any field of medicine, an understanding of the primary goals of care are essential to effective practice.

2.1.1 Anatomy

The upper extremity includes structures from the shoulder to the tips of the fingers. Historically, "arm" refers to the region from the shoulder to the elbow, whereas "forearm" refers to the region from the elbow to the wrist. The majority of pathology in the esports population occurs more distally in the forearm. Subsequently, proximal structures will be touched on only briefly.

The upper extremity consists of a total of 64 bones, with 10 in the shoulder and arm, 16 in the wrist, and 38 in the hand. The humerus of the arm articulates with the radius and ulna at the elbow joint. The medial and lateral epicondyles of the humerus are prominent anatomical structures that serve as attachment points for muscles of the distal arm.

The medial epicondyle is more prominent than its lateral component and serves as a major attachment point for flexors and pronators of the forearm. It also protects the ulnar nerve with a groove along the posterior side. The lateral epicondyle serves as an attachment point for extensors and supinators.

The radius and ulna are connected by a fibrous interosseous membrane. Distally, they articulate with respective carpal bones of the hand. At the wrist, the extensor tendons are separated by six anatomical tunnels called compartments, which are shown in Fig. 2.1 and described in Table 2.1.

The brachial plexus provides the majority of nerve supply to the upper extremity and arises from the anterior rami of the lower four cervical nerves and first thoracic nerve. The plexus forms the major nerves of the upper extremity: the ulnar, median, and radial nerve.

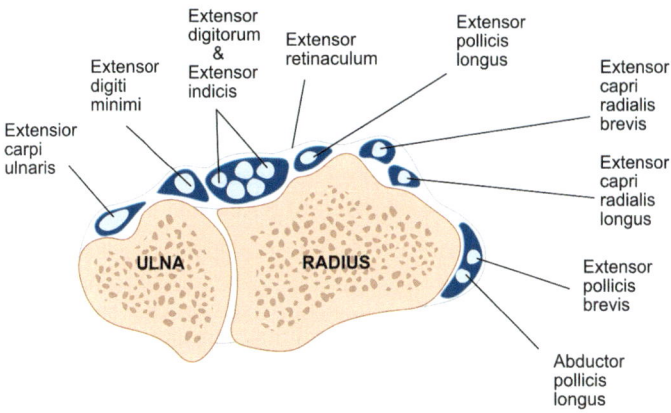

Fig. 2.1 The extensor compartments of the wrist cover the dorsal surface of the radius and ulna, and contain tendons of wrist, finger, and thumb extension, as well as thumb abduction

Table 2.1 The extensor compartments of the wrist components and actions

Compartment	Components	Actions
1	Abductor pollicis longus Extensor pollicis brevis	Thumb abduction Metacarpophalangeal extension
2	Extensor carpi radialis longus and brevis	Wrist extension
3	Extensor pollicis longus	Thumb interphalangeal joint extension
4	Extensor digitorum Extensor indicis	Finger extension
5	Extensor digiti minimi	5th digit extension
6	Extensor carpi ulnaris	Wrist extension and adduction

2.1.2   Evaluation

A challenge that many practitioners in the realm of esports medicine may face is the relative unwillingness or uneasiness to address illnesses affecting the upper extremity. Some degree of discomfort or pain may be considered normal for many who have placed their bodies under such specific stresses for an extended period of time. Thorough knowledge of not only anatomy and pathology but also specific gaming mechanics relevant to the player is essential to proper diagnosis. Furthermore, when pathology is found, examination of the contralateral side is paramount for tests from simple range of motion to electrodiagnostics. This can help eliminate false positive test results and avoid unnecessary interventions.

2.1.2.1 History Taking

Careful history taking is an essential first step, and can often narrow the diagnosis drastically with only a few basic questions. Certain clinical pearls are especially helpful for the esports athlete, and are discussed below.

Location

Where exactly symptoms arise can reveal vast amounts of clinical information. It can be helpful to ask them to use one finger to localize the area, rather than their entire hand. Although not a hard-and-fast rule, ligament and tendon injuries tend to be more easy to localize in that fashion than nerve injuries, which can present more diffusely.

Onset

What was the player doing at the time of injury? A slow, insidious course may have a difficult onset to pinpoint. This may suggest chronic microtraumas or compression as causative factors. An acute onset of symptoms is less common in this patient population. Due to the repetitive strain of gaming, underlying pathological changes may make structures more susceptible to acute injuries. Therefore, acute injuries may be more complicated than originally assumed.

Did the symptoms start with any recent changes in setup, such as a new keyboard or controller? Different keyboard angles and sizes, the addition of paddles, or mouse heights may provoke specific ailments.

Palliation and Provocation

What activities bring on the symptoms? For some, this will most likely be extended gaming sessions. Do specific titles make symptoms worse than others? For example, in more straightforward first-person shooter titles with traditional WASD keybinds, the breadth of finger range of motion is much smaller when compared to games with build mechanics or complicated keybinds.

Furthermore, pain that is worse upon awakening may point towards nerve injuries that are aggravated by immobility in positions assumed while sleeping.

Quality

Although not a hard-and-fast rule, pain that is described as "burning," "electric," and "radiating" may more commonly be associated with nerve injuries whereas words like "sore" and "stabbing" may describe tendon or muscle involvement.

Radiation

Do the symptoms travel? If so, where? Symptoms that travel across two joint lines may point more closely to nerve injuries rather than tendon or muscle involvement. The symptoms may also follow a specific dermatomal or peripheral nerve pattern, further aiding diagnosis.

However, nerve injuries may also be the hardest to pinpoint, and patients may gesture with their entire hand over a specific area, rather than being able to label the exact spot as with conditions like epicondylitis.

Esports History

A careful esports history is also essential, and should include what system the athletes primarily utilizes, what main titles they are playing, training schedule details, and what forms of physical activity are being utilized. As mentioned before, video games drastically differ in mechanics, and may result in a variety of injury patterns.

If possible, a thorough evaluation of the exact keybinds a player is using may reveal an overuse of the affected area. This will also provide valuable insight into possible interventions once a diagnosis is made.

2.1.2.2 Physical Examination

A focused physical examination should include a careful inspection of the involved area, as well as the joints above and below. For a musculoskeletal examination to be complete, it must include inspection, range of motion (both passive and active), palpation, muscle strength testing, and further special testing.

Inspection

Subtle clues and diagnostic details can be glimmered from simple inspection. The area should be completely exposed to allow for thorough evaluation. Inspection can reveal things such as swelling, erythema, and deformity.

Palpation

When palpating a possible area of pain, care should be taken to avoid the area of maximal tenderness until the last possible moment. This will increase the chances of a successful exam. Palpation allows examiners to also feel for areas of tautness, warmth, and effusions.

Range of Motion

Both passive and active range of motion is essential to determining not only pathology, but possible therapeutic interventions. For example, severely restricted wrist flexion due to muscle tightness might not be the presenting symptom, but treatments that focus on improved range of motion may help the underlying diagnosis.

Range of motion testing should also include pinpointing the causative motion, if one exists. A small amount of resistance may be applied to aid diagnosis.

Sensory Examination

A basic understanding of peripheral nerve distribution (Fig. 2.2), as well as dermatomes, is essential to effective physical examination. Of importance, there exists a great deal of sensory redundancy

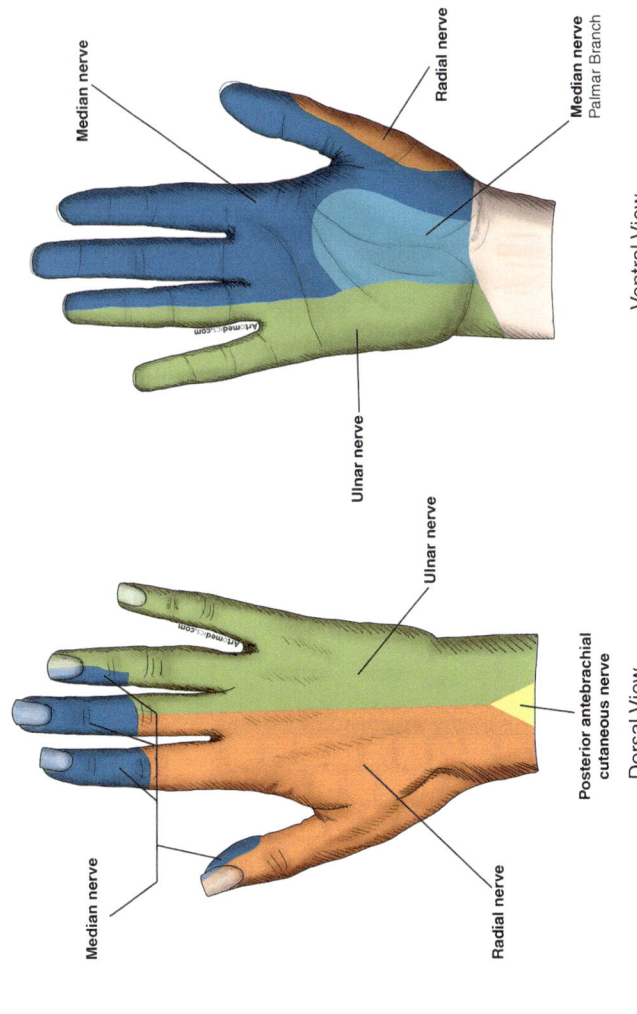

Fig. 2.2 Cutaneous innervation of the hand via peripheral nerves

in the upper extremity. This overlapping of nerve distributions can often confound the examination.

Motor Examination

Manual muscle testing can be performed to establish strength and also reveal areas of imbalance. It is important to realize that in gamers hand dominance might mean less in terms of side-to-side differences. For example, in the normal population, the dominant hand may have a relative strength in finger abduction. However, for a right-handed PC gamer who utilizes the "Tab," "Caps Lock," and "Shift" keys more frequently (Fig. 2.3), the left side may in fact be stronger. This could be an important differentiator between a clinical suggestion of cubital tunnel syndrome and a simple key-bind explanation.

Another important point is that pain in a specific tendon or joints can result in give-way weakness, and should be appropriately documented [1].

Tinel's Test

The Tinel's test is a technique used to detect nerve inflammation, and can be applied to multiple anatomical locations. To perform, light percussion is applied to a nerve. The test is considered positive if paresthesia is elicited in the nerve's distribution.

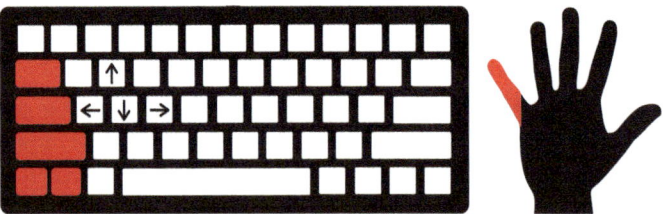

Fig. 2.3 Aerial keyboard view with buttons most commonly accessed using the fifth digit. These keys are often bound to frequently used actions such as crouch, inventory, map, sprint, or special attacks. The fifth digit is persistently utilized for these actions as the second to fourth digits are usually engaged in movement, thus leaving only the first and fifth digits readily available

2.1.2.3 Imaging

Ultrasonography

Musculoskeletal ultrasound (US) can be one of the most useful imaging techniques when approached correctly in the hands of a skilled clinician, so much so that it can be considered an extension of the physical examination. Examiners trained correctly can not only obtain real-time, dynamic images of involved structures, but offer more precise interventions. Other advantages include absence of radiation exposure, ease of accessibility, patient involvement, and cost-effectiveness.

A variety of transducers, also known as probes, are available. The most commonly used probes for the evaluation of the upper extremity are the linear and small-footprint linear array. Linear probes are more commonly used for superficial anatomy such as the tendons and nerves of the hand and wrist. The small-footprint linear array probe, also known as the hockey-stick transducer for its characteristic appearance has a higher frequency, and can provide a higher image resolution for the most superficial of structures.

A basic understanding of US terminology is essential for every clinician who wishes to understand and effectively treat esports conditions. The fundamentals of US comes from a structure's echogenicity, that is, how strongly a structure reflects the transducer's sound wave. A hyperechoic structure (with high echogenicity) will strongly reflect the sound of the ultrasound back at the transducer. This increased signal will result in the structure appearing bright on US. Hyperechoic structures include tendons and the outer surfaces of bone. On the contrary, a hypoechoic structure will appear darker, and denotes a lower density. Anechoic structures will appear black and do not reflect any sound waves. Fluid is the most relevant anechoic substance. In reality, most structures are a mixture of echogenicity based on their underlying heterogeneity. For example, a peripheral nerve consists of hypoechoic individual nerve fascicles surrounded by hyperechoic epineurium.

A thorough examination includes evaluation of the structure in both short axis and long axis. This allows for not only correct identification of structures, but more complete analysis for pathology. In the long axis, a nerve may appear similar to surrounding tendons, but on short axis, the characteristic "honey-comb" appearance is difficult to confuse. Practitioners who wish to learn more about ultrasonography as a diagnostic tool are encouraged to refer to dedicated handbooks [2].

Radiography
X-ray has limited value in a variety of these cases, aside from ruling out a more insidious cause. If the history lacks a traumatic event, x-ray is rarely indicated.

Magnetic Resonance Imaging
While Magnetic Resonance Imaging (MRI) has the advantage of lack of radiation exposure and thorough evaluation of soft tissue structures, it can be costly and oftentimes unnecessary. However, when the diagnosis is uncertain after thorough physical examination and ultrasound, MRI may be necessary. T1-weighted images provide the best resolution for examining anatomy, whereas T2-weighted images can demonstrate the presence of fluid or cysts [3].

> **Clinical Pearl**
> When Triangular Fibrocartilage Complex involvement is suspected, MRI is an essential diagnostic tool.

Electrodiagnostics
In a trained hand, electrodiagnostics (EDX) can provide vital information concerning possible neuromuscular disorders. They are best considered extensions of a thorough neurological examination, rather than separate tests on their own. Given the intense technicality and choice of study parameters based on individualized clinical decision making, diagnostics should be approached only after a thorough differential diagnosis has been formed.

These studies can include a multitude of techniques, but for the scope of this textbook we will discuss nerve conduction studies (NCS) and needle electromyography (EMG).

NCSs are performed by placing recording surface electrodes over the motor or sensory innervation of a specific nerve. The corresponding peripheral nerve is then stimulated proximally, and the motor and sensory responses are recorded. The responses are known as compound muscle action potentials (CMAPs) and sensory nerve action potentials (SNAPs), respectively. Furthermore, the speed of impulse transmission can also be quantified as "conduction velocity". These values can then be compared to standardized numbers to evaluate for neuropathic and myopathic lesions, as well as disorders of the neuromuscular junction. When abnormal values are found, contralateral investigation is strongly recommended to rule out congenital or anomalous abnormalities [4].

EMG utilizes a needle electrode placed directly within the muscle, allowing for individual motor unit examination. It is often more challenging and places the patient in a higher level of discomfort than NCS. Any provider who refers a patient for an EDX should warn their patient at that time that the test involves needle examination of the involved area and may cause them discomfort [5].

EDX can be helpful in pinpointing disorders of the peripheral nervous system, which are all too common in the gaming population. Poor ergonomics, hypertonicity, and prolonged compression is an environment ripe for nerve compression and damage.

2.1.3   Treatment

2.1.3.1 Therapeutic Modalities

The most common modality utilized by patients prior to presentation is by far cold therapy. Cold therapy can reduce pain via vasoconstriction, decreased inflammation and metabolic demand [6]. Nontraditional modalities, such as acupuncture, yoga, and osteopathic manual therapy, may also be helpful for certain cases.

Kinesio tape is an elastic therapeutic skin tape thought to act by providing support to muscles and joints, thus allowing for continued movements with decreased pain. Current evidence is mixed for the role of kinesiotaping, but it may be beneficial for certain conditions [7, 8].

2.1.3.2 Rehabilitation
Referral to an occupational therapist or certified hand therapist can allow patients to take a more active role in their recovery. When weakness is present on physical examination, this referral becomes more than necessary. Even with the most motivated of populations, self-directed programs may not be as regular or effective as a formal course of therapy.

2.1.3.3 Pharmacology
Over-the-counter medications such as nonsteroidal anti-inflammatory drugs (NSAIDs) and acetaminophen may provide temporary pain relief in acute phases. NSAIDs such as ibuprofen and naproxen block the inflammatory cascade via inhibiting the activity of cyclooxygenase enzymes (COX 1 and/or 2). Long-term NSAID usage can have deleterious effects, such as gastrointestinal distress/damage and kidney dysfunction. NSAIDs may also interact with other medication metabolism. Topical NSAIDs can provide pain relief for some of the more superficial structures while circumventing the deleterious adverse effects.

Anticonvulsants and antidepressants have been proven effective for certain painful conditions. Neuropathic causes, such as peripheral nerve entrapments, with symptoms of paresthesia and dysesthesia may respond to such agents. It is important to educate patients that these medications will have little effect on numbness [9].

2.1.3.4 Interventions
For cases unresponsive to conservative management, further intervention may be necessary. Nerve blocks, regenerative medicine injections, and corticosteroid injections should always be performed under ultrasound guidance for greater efficacy and avoidance of adverse effects. Steroid injections are not recommended for long-term use due to the deleterious effects on healthy cartilage, bones, and tendons.

2.2   Hand and Wrist

2.2.1   Radial Styloid Tenosynovitis

De Quervain's Tenosynovitis, Gamer's Thumb, Selfie Thumb, Falcon Thumb, Mommy's Thumb

2.2.1.1 Overview

With the advent of the smartphone, this clinical syndrome previously associated with new parents has risen to prominence in the public eye. Radial styloid tenosynovitis is characterized by pain in the radial wrist, specifically during thumb or wrist movement.

2.2.1.2 Pathogenesis

The first compartment of the wrist is composed of the extensor pollicis brevis (EPB) and abductor pollicis longus (APL). Combined, their actions work to bring the thumb away from the palm in abduction and extension.

> **Clinical Pearl**
> A useful mnemonic for remembering the involved tendons in this condition is "All Peanut Lovers Eat Peanut Butter".

Both the APL and EPB lie in a fibrous sheath within the synovial lining. This sheath crosses the radial styloid and passes under the extensor retinaculum. Cadaverous examination has revealed that there may be a small septa separating the two, or they may have entirely different synovial sheaths. The presence of a septum is thought to increase the risk of developing radial styloid tenosynovitis, and may have clinical treatment implications which will be discussed later [10].

Repetitive trauma such as chronic overuse or rapid increase in usage places shear forces on the tendons resulting in thickening and tenosynovitis. Positions that increase the stress on the tendons, such as extension and abduction, are thought to lead to an increased risk of injury.

Despite being described as a stenosing tenosynovitis, which describes an inflammation of the synovial sheath of a tendon, this description is not entirely accurate. Histopathological evaluation of patients who were treated surgically for radial styloid tenosynovitis have shown the process is noninflammatory in nature and instead a degenerative process [11].

2.2.1.3 Presentation

Nonspecific pain in the radial wrist is a common presenting symptom. Pain may radiate into the thumb or down the forearm, and can be described as sharp or burning. Symptoms are often aggravated by thumb or wrist movement, including rotatory and gripping movements, and when using a controller's analog stick. With advanced disease, patients may complain of weakness with grip. With most overuse injuries, the onset is often gradual with no clear defined onslaught.

2.2.1.4 Diagnosis

This is largely a clinical diagnosis with no advanced imaging required for uncomplicated cases. Although there are no high-quality clinical studies on the subject, the authors speculate this is more common in controller players than PC, given bilateral thumb positioning.

Physical Examination

Inspection may reveal mild swelling overlying the radial styloid or just proximal, and palpation of the area may elicit pain. Precise location is helpful when determining if the patient's lateral wrist pain is due to radial styloid tenosynovitis or intersection syndrome.

Clinical Pearl
Symptoms from radial styloid tenosynovitis is more commonly distal and lateral, whereas intersection syndrome presents more dorsal and proximal.

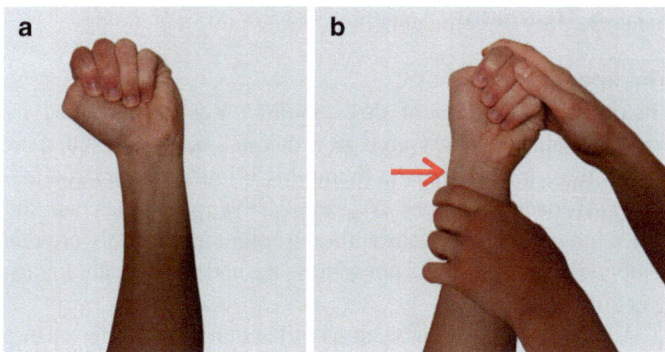

Fig. 2.4 Finkelstein's test. (**a**) Patients place their thumb inside of a closed fist. (**b**) The examiner then stabilizes the forearm with one hand, and ulnarly deviates the patient's hand with the other. The arrow corresponds to the most common area of pain, and signifies a positive test

Finkelstein's Test

This test can often be diagnostic if performed correctly. As shown in Fig. 2.4, patients are instructed to grasp their thumb in their palm, and close their fist. The examiner then stabilizes the forearm with one hand, and ulnarly deviates the patient's hand with the other. Reproduction of pain over the EPB and APL signifies a positive test, and is usually diagnostic of radial styloid tenosynovitis. As many gamers and non-gamers may have never stretched these muscles before, tightness should be expected and may not correlate with injury.

Imaging

Imaging is usually not necessary, but ultrasound can confirm the diagnosis if the differential is still broad. Ultrasonographic evaluation can reveal thickening of the suspected tendons. A thin echogenic line between the APL and EPB tendons signifies the presence of a septum, which may predispose a patient to tenosynovitis [12].

2.2.1.5 Treatment

Therapeutic Modalities

Historically, treatment of this condition was accompanied by immobilization of the thumb in a thumb spica splint. Of note, splints must immobilize the thumb MCP joint in order to effectively off-load the tendons in question. However, as the condition is not inflammatory in nature, thumb splinting may only provide temporary pain relief, and not address the underlying pathological process.

Activity modification, such as utilization of a shorter analog stick, can decrease thumb extension and abduction and subsequently decrease stress on the involved tendons. For PC games, a knowledge of a patient's keybinds on the affected side can often aid in prevention.

After pain has subsided, a comprehensive therapy program that involves strengthening exercises, with a special focus on eccentrics and progressive tendon loading, can help adopt a more conducive tendon architecture.

The mainstay of treatment is a combination of thumb spica splint wearing schedules coupled with targeted exercises. Further, kinesiotape can help further stabilize and decompress the joint while performing aggravating activities.

Common concentric and eccentric strengthening exercises include wrist extension/flexion, radial/ulnar deviation, thumb isometric holds, as well as thumb and pinch variations. Exercises can be done with or without weight and should not be done in excess or to the point where pain is felt.

Pharmacological Management

Oral NSAIDs may provide temporary, symptomatic relief but should be avoided for long-term treatment.

Interventional Medicine

For cases not controlled with oral medications and rehabilitation, further interventions may be necessary. Corticosteroid injection can be effective for around 50% of patients, and should always be done under ultrasound guidance. If a septum or separate synovial sheaths are found, multiple sites may need to be injected in order to provide effective treatment [13].

Surgical release may be the final option for the most advanced cases. The first dorsal compartment sheath is opened longitudinally, thus completely releasing the tendons. While this has been shown to be effective, damage to the radial sensory nerve can result [14].

2.2.2   Intersection Syndrome

Proximal Intersection Syndrome, Crossover Syndrome

2.2.2.1 Overview
Often initially misdiagnosed as radial styloid tenosynovitis, intersection syndrome is caused by aggravation of the first and second dorsal muscle compartments at their intersection point.

2.2.2.2 Pathogenesis
The first dorsal compartment of the wrist containing the abductor pollicis longus (APL) and the extensor pollicis brevis (EPB) crosses over the muscle bellies of the second compartment of the wrist containing the extensor carpi radialis longus (ECRL) and brevis (ECRB) tendons. This occurs approximately 4 cm proximal to Lister's tubercle. The ECRL and ECRB largely function in wrist extension, whereas the APL and EPB are responsible for thumb abduction and extension.

With repetitive wrist extension, friction can develop between the two compartments at their crossing point and stimulate an inflammatory response. With continued aggravation, tenosynovitis can develop in one or both compartments. This is more commonly seen when the hand is held in a gripped position and then subjected to flexion and extension, but can occur in a multitude of cases such as PC players with distant thumb keybinds or console players [15].

2.2.2.3 Presentation

The presenting symptom is often dorsal wrist and distal forearm pain overlying the area of intersection, which is proximal and dorsal to the radial styloid. Patients may also describe a sensation or sound of "squeaking" during movements that elicit pain. This sound is unique to intersection syndrome, and its presence should place this diagnosis at the top of the differential.

2.2.2.4 Diagnosis

Intersection syndrome is primarily a clinical diagnosis. The largest diagnostic hurdle is often differentiating it from radial styloid tenosynovitis.

Physical Examination

Palpation may elicit tenderness over the site of intersection, and a small amount of swelling may be visible. Active range of motion testing may reveal crepitus when performing the respective muscle actions, which are wrist and thumb extension. Of note, the presence of crepitus should move intersection syndrome to the top of the differential diagnosis. Resisted extension and supination may reproduce pain in the same distribution.

Imaging

If further diagnostics are needed aside from history and physical examination, bedside ultrasound should be the first step. The most common finding is peritendinous edema. Instead of the usual hyperechoic plane separating the tendons, a hypoechoic area of tendon sheath fluid may be present, signifying underlying tenosynovitis. If the process is chronic, tendon thickening may also be present [16].

2.2.2.5 Treatment

A temporary period of rest and recovery, conservative management focusing on activity modification, and therapeutic exercises are usually sufficient for treatment. However, for recalcitrant cases, further intervention may be necessary.

Once the diagnosis of intersection syndrome is made, the laterality offers further insight. With console controls, the wrist is usually relatively stable, so thumb movement may be a less common cause. If a patient's keyboard hand is affected, careful examination of the height and wrist angle while gaming should be noted and adjusted appropriately. The ergonomics of gaming will be discussed in detail in Chap. 5.

Therapeutic Modalities

Given the superficial nature of the structures, ice may provide temporary pain relief as well as aid in reducing swelling. There are not currently well-established guidelines for rehabilitation of this condition, but referral to a hand therapist should be considered for all patients who do not respond to above treatments. Supervised wrist and thumb strengthening exercises, along with tendon glides and stretches can aid in both prevention and recovery.

Pharmacological Management

Oral anti-inflammatories may provide temporary pain relief and should be avoided in the long term. Topical anti-inflammatories may also be of use, given the superficial structures and inflammatory nature of the disorder.

Interventional Medicine

When conservative management fails, corticosteroid injections under ultrasound guidance can be a logical next step. In rare cases, surgical debridement and release involving the release of the second dorsal compartment can provide relief [17].

Intersection Syndrome Versus Radial Styloid Tenosynovitis
Both involve the first compartment of the wrist, but intersection syndrome occurs more proximally, where the first compartment crosses over the second. Subsequently, pain from intersection syndrome will be more dorsal, and radial styloid tenosynovitis pain more radial, as shown in Fig. 2.5. Crepitus has only been reported in intersection syndrome, and is historically absent in radial styloid tenosynovitis.

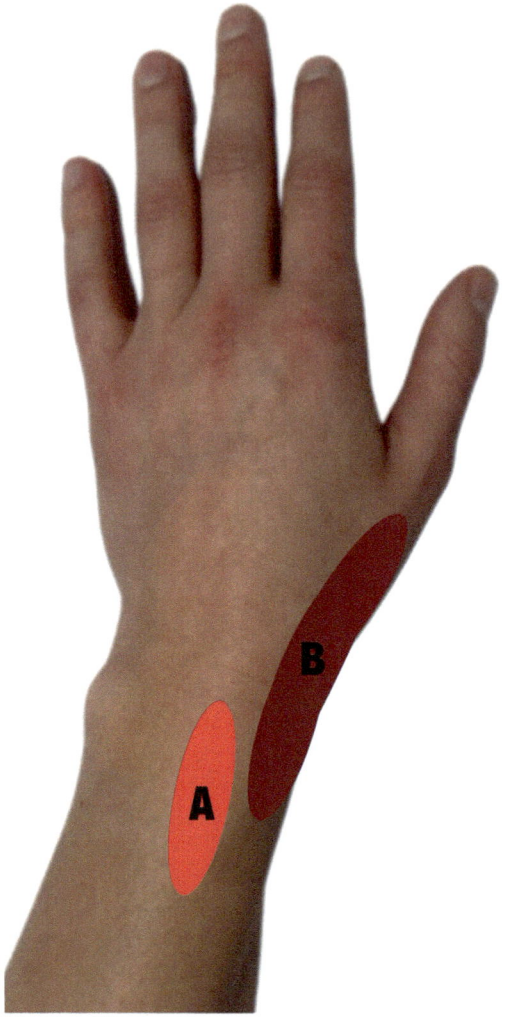

Fig. 2.5 Common locations for pain for (**a**) intersection syndrome and (**b**) radial styloid tenosynovitis

2.2.3 Extensor Carpi Ulnaris Tendonitis

2.2.3.1 Overview

The Extensor Carpi Ulnaris (ECU) is a thin muscle located in the posterior compartment of the forearm. Injury, usually secondary to repetitive or forceful wrist movement, results in ulnar-sided hand, wrist and forearm pain.

2.2.3.2 Pathogenesis

The ECU originates from the distal humerus as part of the common extensor tendon and inserts on the base of the fifth metacarpal base. The tendon enters an osteofibrous sheath at the head of the ulna that passes deep to the extensor retinaculum prior to its insertion. Fascia overlies the osseous groove, forming the ECU subsheath. This is unique to the ECU when compared to the extensor compartments. The action depends on the position of the forearm, with extension and adduction of the wrist being predominant. It also contributes to medial wrist stability.

Pathology can arise proximally or distally, the former being discussed later in the chapter in "Lateral epicondylitis." Distal pathology arises from the unique anatomy of the ECU when compared to the other extensor tendons.

The ECU is much more restricted in movement than the other extensor tendons, due in part to its separate subsheath which places varying amounts of stress depending on wrist positioning. Unlike the extensor retinaculum, which runs from the radius to carpal bones, and thus is not affected by supination or pronation, the subsheath has an ulnar attachment and thus varies with the aforementioned positions.

With the wrist held in pronation, the angle of the ECU tendon as it exits the subsheath is approximately neutral. During supination, the ECU bends at the subsheath, reaching an angle of approximately 30° prior to attachment on its insertion point, as shown in Fig. 2.6. This also places the ECU in close proximity to the extensor digiti minimi and subjects it to maximal traction [18].

The ECU tendon sheath can be irritated by repetitive wrist movements, most commonly dorsiflexion and rotation of the

Fig. 2.6 With the forearm in pronation, the extensor carpi ulnaris (ECU) tendon exits its subsheath with a relative neutral angle. However, when the forearm is supinated and flexed when holding a controller, the tendon bends as it exits the subsheath

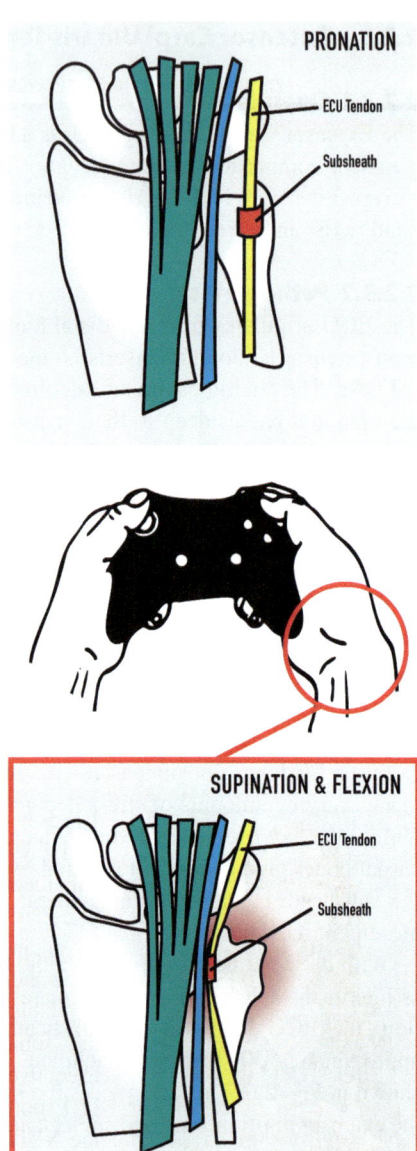

wrist. Pain often develops where the tendon bends as it exits the fibro-osseous tunnel on the ulna. While ECU tendonitis is more commonly found in racket sports or following a Colles' fracture, esports athletes are uniquely susceptible to injuries of this thin muscle.

Non-neutral wrist positioning on keyboards or computer mice, such as dorsiflexion, places the tendon under increased and constant stress. Rapid wrist adduction, often required for "flick shots" and reaching more lateral keybinds, causes further microtrauma. Similarly, gaming controllers are often held with a partially supinated, flexed, and ulnarly deviated wrist, when the ECU is under maximal stress.

With untreated and undiagnosed tendonitis, more serious tendinopathy can gradually develop. In rare cases, complications such as subluxation may occur. Subluxation occurs most commonly when the ECU is isometrically contracting with the wrist held in a position of supination, flexion and ulnar deviation, coupled with the application of a sudden force. Although this situation would be outside of the realm of normal esports, an accidental force being applied to a player's hand while they are holding a controller could theoretically result in such an injury [19].

2.2.3.3 Presentation

Patients with distal ECU tendonitis will often complain of dorsal, ulnar-sided wrist pain. Unless there was a presenting trauma, such as a fall or fracture, onset is most often insidious. Specific motions, such as ulnar deviation in extension, may worsen pain. "Keyboard holidays," that is, extended periods of time not at their desk or setup, may result in alleviation of pain. In more advanced cases, patients may complain of loss of grip strength. If subluxation concurrently exists, patients may describe a sensation of clicking or popping as the wrist is actively moved into extension and supination.

2.2.3.4 Diagnosis

Upon presentation, the clinical picture of ECU tendonitis may be hard to differentiate from injury to the triangular fibrocartilage complex (TFCC). Given the drastic difference in management, proper diagnostic procedures are necessary for successful outcomes.

Physical Examination

Due to the superficial nature of the ECU, slight swelling of the ulnar sheath may be visible, and palpation can easily locate the tendon. Patients with longstanding damage may have tenderness more proximally, up the length of the muscle, despite no subjective complaints of proximal symptoms.

Depending on acuity, passive and active wrist extension and ulnar deviation may elicit discomfort. Similarly, resisted isometric supination can also provoke symptoms. Traditionally, resisted extension and ulnar deviation was used to diagnose ECU pathology. However, this position similarly loads the TFCC and is of little clinical value.

Special testing can be the most useful to diagnose this clinical syndrome.

ECU Synergy Test

The patient rests their arm on the examination table with the elbow flexed to 90° and the forearm held in maximal supination. The position of the wrist is neutral, and the fingers are in full extension. The examiner then grasps the patient's thumb and index finger with one hand, while the other hand locates the ECU tendon. The patient then actively radially abducts the thumb against examiner's resistance. The examiner confirms engagement of the ECU muscle contraction. Re-creation of pain along the dorsal ulnar aspect of the wrist is considered to be a positive test for ECU tendonitis [20].

Imaging

Under ultrasound, the ECU is easily identified as it is the most superficial muscle on the ulnar side of the forearm. Ultrasound also offers the option of dynamic examination with supination and pronation. Peritendinous edema is usually present, with some degree of tendon thickening. For long-standing or severe cases, intratendon tears may be visualized.

For refractory cases or when the differential is still uncertain, MRI can be utilized to properly visualize the involved structures.

2.2.3.5 Treatment

Attention should be paid to a gamer's keyboard, focusing on wrist neutrality in all planes. Bulky mechanical keyboards can place the wrist into extension, increasing tension in the ECU. A decreased keyboard slope has been associated with decreased activation of the ECU [21].

Therapeutic Modalities

Splinting may be temporarily beneficial to reduce inflammation and pain. Splints that reduce radial and ulnar deviation are often chosen, with some placing the wrist in 30° of extension. Current literature suggests duration of use for approximately 4 weeks with removal for therapy. Exercises with light resistance and weight, as well as isometric holds can be performed to increase endurance and strength of affected musculature. Incorporating tendon and ulnar nerve glides may also be performed for further prevention and treatment.

Pharmacological Management

Oral and topical NSAIDs may be helpful for inflammation reduction and pain relief in the acute phases.

Interventional Medicine

For refractory symptoms or when immediate pain relief is necessary, a targeted corticosteroid injection to the area of dysfunction may provide relief. To ensure accuracy, ultrasound guidance is recommended. However, this may increase risk of tendon rupture, an uncommon but serious complication. In rare cases, surgical repair on the tendon and its sheath may be necessary [22].

2.2.4   Median Neuropathy at the Wrist

Carpal tunnel syndrome

2.2.4.1 Overview

The median nerve is one of five main upper extremity nerves arising from the brachial plexus. It has multiple sensory and motor innervations, and is essential for proper upper extremity functioning. Nontraumatic compression of the median nerve can arise in multiple locations, such as the pronator teres and carpal tunnel of the wrist. Carpal tunnel syndrome (CTS) results from compression of the median nerve as it enters the hand inside of the carpal tunnel. This clinical syndrome results in tingling and numbness in a stereotypical distribution, as well as hand weakness. CTS is the most common nerve entrapment in the upper extremity.

2.2.4.2 Pathogenesis

The carpal tunnel describes an anatomic compartment of the proximal hand that can be approximated superficially at the level of the distal wrist crease. It is bordered by carpal bones on three sides, and the transverse carpal ligament on the anterior side. The transverse carpal ligament is a fibrous band that runs medially from the pisiform laterally to the hamate, and is also known as the flexor retinaculum. The carpal tunnel contains nine flexor tendons and the median nerve.

The median nerve is responsible for sensory innervation of the palmar surface of the thumb, index, middle finger, and lateral half of the ring finger, as well as the thenar eminence. It provides motor innervation to the flexor pollicis brevis, abductor pollicis brevis, and opponens pollicis, which are responsible for thumb flexion, abduction, and opposition.

Being bound on three sides by bones and a fourth by a tough fibrous structure, the size of the carpal tunnel is relatively fixed. Similarly, the compressibility of the flexors tendons is inconsequential compared to that of the median nerve. As a result, when space becomes sparse inside the canal, the median nerve is the first to suffer. Canal space can be decreased by a variety of intrinsic or extrinsic factors, but most pertinent to the gaming population is via swelling or thickening of the flexor tendons and wrist positioning.

Wrist positioning is an exceptionally important consideration for PC gamers. While a neutral wrist is optimal, due to large mechanical keyboards and thicker gaming mice the wrist is often held to some degree of extension. With wrist movements outside of neutral, carpal tunnel pressures have been measured almost 10 times that of normal [23, 24].

Mild compression can lead to a physiologic conduction block. This early nerve injury is usually completely recoverable as the endoneurium, perineurium, and epineurium are intact. However, with longstanding, repetitive damage myelin and the surrounding connective tissue framework may be disrupted, resulting in irreversible damage.

2.2.4.3 Presentation
Numbness and tingling in the sensory distribution of the median nerve are often the first signs of CTS. Sensation to the thenar eminence and palm is spared, as the palmar cutaneous branch of the median nerve arises in the distal forearm, and does not traverse the carpal tunnel. Patients will complain of paresthesia which are often worse at night or upon awakening. This is often due to accentuated and sustained wrist flexion or extension while asleep. Neuropathic pain may accompany sensory disturbances, and it is not uncommon for patients to complain of symptoms proximal to the carpal tunnel. However, paresthesias that radiate into the neck should raise suspicion for an alternative diagnosis.

Long-standing compression can lead to weakness in the muscles innervated by the median nerve. This can manifest as difficulty reaching keybinds on the right side of the keyboard, weakness when holding the controller, handwriting changes, difficulty with opening jars, or dropping cups.

2.2.4.4 Diagnosis
There is no standardized set of diagnostic criteria for median neuropathy, but rather a constellation of symptoms and clinical findings. Electrophysiological testing can be quite useful.

Physical Examination

Inspection of the hands may reveal thenar eminence atrophy, which is a sign of severe, longstanding CTS. Sensory examination can elicit decreased sensation of the first three digits and stereotypical splitting of the ring finger. Examiners can compare the medial, ulnarly innervated side of the ring finger to the lateral, median innervated side. Weakness in the median innervated muscles can be found on motor testing, which are the flexor pollicis brevis, opponens pollicis, and abductor pollicis brevis. A variety of special testing also aids in clinical diagnosis.

> **Clinical Pearl**
> The median innervated hand muscles can be easily recollected using the LOAF acronym: Lumbricals 1 and 2, Opponens pollicis, Abductor pollicis brevis, Flexor pollicis brevis.

Phalen's Maneuver

The patient's wrists are placed into full flexion for a total of 60 s. While this is often taught with patient's in the "reverse prayer pose," the authors encourage extending the elbows forward as well. This avoids aggravation of any underlying cubital tunnel syndrome with elbow flexion, thus confounding the results.

Carpal Compression Test

This test is performed by placing sustained direct pressure over the volar aspect of the wrist, directly over the carpal tunnel, for at least 30 s. The pressure can be held for up to 2 min.

Both Phalen's test and the carpal compression test are considered positive if paresthesia is generated in the distribution of the median nerve. These tests can be combined, as in Fig. 2.7, by placing compression over the median nerve while the patient's wrists are held in complete flexion.

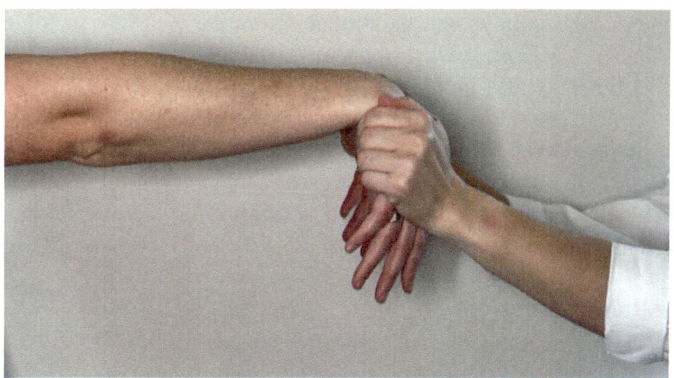

Fig. 2.7 Combined Phalen's Maneuver and Carpal Compression Test

Tinel's at Wrist
To address the median nerve, light percussion is applied to the midline of the distal palmar crease. The test is considered positive if paresthesia is elicited in the first three digits.

Imaging
Ultrasound can be used to visualize the median nerve in the carpal tunnel. The presence of median nerve enlargement proximal to the carpal tunnel suggests a diagnosis of CTS.

Electrodiagnostics
Electrodiagnostics (EDX) may aid in diagnosis, but findings should not be taken in isolation. Up to 15% of patients with clinically diagnosed CTS may have normal EDX findings. Furthermore, severity of CTS symptoms does not always correlate with EDX findings.

Sensory nerve conduction studies (NCS) are more sensitive than motor findings given their susceptibility to compression and ischemia. NCS will reveal slowing or a conduction block of the median nerve fibers across the carpal tunnel. EMG evaluation is targeted towards needle evaluation of the abductor pollicis brevis (APB). The APB may not be involved in mild cases of CTS, and thus EMG findings will be normal. However, with longstanding damage, EMG may reveal signs of axonal loss.[5]

EDX may also be used for severity grading. One of the most widely accepted neurophysiological grading scales is the Bland criteria, and ranks CTS from grade 0 (normal) to grade 6 (extremely severe). These grading scales may be helpful in selecting appropriate treatments, such as informing outcomes when deciding on surgical interventions [25, 26].

2.2.4.5 Treatment

Therapeutic Modalities
Treatment for mild cases begins with nocturnal wrist splinting. Most over-the-counter braces place the wrist in mild extension, which may need to be corrected. Other treatments include the use of kinesio tape during the day when performing repetitive tasks which is hypothesized to increase stability and off-load the carpal tunnel to relieve pain.

Targeted occupational therapy includes median nerve glides and tendon glides, allowing for tendons and nerves to freely pass through the carpal tunnel. General wrist strengthening in pain-free movements can help increase wrist endurance. Manual therapy, mainly gradual gentle to deep massage of the forearm performed by a trained therapist, may also prove to be beneficial.

Pharmacological Management
For patients experiencing primarily neuropathic pain, gabapentin and other nerve medications can provide relief.

Interventional Medicine
An ultrasound-guided corticosteroid injection can be used to treat mild CTS symptoms. Severe cases that exhibit overt muscle atrophy or failure of conservative treatment most often require surgical release of the flexor retinaculum. However, patients with long-standing disease should be counselled that numbness and weakness may never resolve.

2.2.5 Triangular Fibrocartilage Complex Injury

Ulnar Impaction Syndrome

2.2.5.1 Overview

The triangular fibrocartilage complex (TFCC) stabilizes the wrist and can be conceptualized as a homologue of the knee's meniscus. While TFCC injuries in esports athletes are extremely rare, given the urgent need for intervention and similarity with ECU tendonitis, it warrants a brief mention.

2.2.5.2 Pathogenesis

The TFCC is composed of the triangular fibrocartilage disc, radioulnar ligaments, and ulnocarpal ligaments. The primary function of the TFCC is load transmission across the ulnocarpal joint, and stabilization of the distal radioulnar joint and ulnocarpal articulations.

The TFCC is the most commonly injured traumatically, with the wrist in extension and pronation and an axial load is applied. This is often seen after a fall on the outstretched hand. Degenerative tears are often seen in athletics and professions that rely on hand function, such as golfers, gymnasts, carpenters, and plumbers. As such, the latter can be extrapolated to be relevant to the gaming population.

Ulnar variance, the relative distance between the articular surfaces of the distal radius and ulna, plays a large part in the load transmission from the wrist through the distal ulna. With increased ulnar variance, the load placed upon the TFCC increases. Similarly, wrist pronation also increases TFCC load [27].

2.2.5.3 Presentation

The primary symptom of a TFCC injury is often pain along the ulnar wrist, just distal to the ulnar styloid. Movements such as rotation (supination and pronation) and ulnar deviation often aggravate pain. Patients may frequently complain of pain when turning a door key or from using their hands to rise from a seated position. Other symptoms such as ulnar-sided wrist swelling, loss of grip strength, and crepitus may also be reported [28].

2.2.5.4 Diagnosis

Physical Examination

Palpation in the soft spot between the ulnar styloid and flexor carpi ulnaris tendon may evoke tenderness, which is known as a positive "fovea" sign.

Symptoms may also be provoked by compressing the joint with an axial load. This is performed by holding the forearm with one hand and placing the wrist in a position of ulnar deviation and extension with the other, subsequently compressing the joint.

Imaging

Plain anteroposterior radiographs are only useful if the etiology is traumatic or to calculate ulnar variance. MRI arthrography may be utilized if the diagnosis is unclear, and can detect TFCC tears on T1-weighted imaging. Fluid may also appear in the distal radioulnar joint. Arthroscopy is the most accurate method of diagnosis.

Ultrasonographic evaluation of the TFCC can be challenging. It normally appears as a hyperechoic triangular-shaped structure that comes into contact with the triquetrum. Injury may be represented as subtly as abnormal hypoechogenicity, thinning, or absence entirely [29].

2.2.5.5 Treatment

Therapeutic Modalities

For mild cases with no wrist instability, a TFCC splint can be utilized for a duration of 4 weeks. General wrist, grip, and forearm strengthening exercises, along with stretching can help reduce the risk of injury [30].

Interventional Medicine

If pain persists beyond 4 weeks, referral to a hand surgeon may be necessary. Similarly, if MRI reveals injury to the central articular disc of the TFCC or if wrist instability is present, surgery is the treatment of choice [31].

2.2.6   Thumb Carpometacarpal Arthritis

2.2.6.1 Overview

Osteoarthritis of the first carpometacarpal (CMC) joint is a common disease in patients over the age of 50. However, due to the increased use and pressures placed on the gamer's thumb, this pathology may have a higher prevalence in the younger esports population.

2.2.6.2 Pathogenesis

The CMC joint is a saddle joint created by the articulation of the first metacarpal with the trapezium bone. It lacks bony confinement, placing increased importance on the surrounding ligaments for stabilization. The anterior ligament, known as the beak ligament, is the most important stabilizer. Laxity of the beak ligament can lead to increased stress loads on the CMC joint.

2.2.6.3 Presentation

Patients often complain of diffuse thumb pain that is typically difficult to localize. It may be aggravated by positions that require sustained flexion, such as use of a controller, buttoning, pinching, grasping, or turning a key. Swelling, stiffness, crepitus, and weakness may also be presenting symptoms.

2.2.6.4 Diagnosis

Physical Examination

Inspection can reveal metacarpal base enlargement, resulting in a visible deformity. Palpation of the volar aspect of the CMC joint usually elicits tenderness. Strength testing may reveal weakness in thumb flexion that is due to pain and disuse rather than inherent muscle weakness.

Grind Test

Axial load is placed on the CMC joint from the distal thumb, while introducing slight rotation. A positive test is signified by pain or crepitus.

Imaging

X-ray reveals early findings of osteoarthritis, such as joint space narrowing. With longer-standing cases, later signs of osteoarthritis such as osteophytes, subchondral sclerosis, and cysts may be present [32].

2.2.6.5 Treatment

Given the younger patient population in esports, treatment should largely focus on prevention of CMC injury. While there is a lack of relevant data on this specific injury in our target population, understanding of the pathophysiology points towards a probable future prevalence.

Osteoarthritis of any joint is largely irreversible. However, with rehabilitation and symptom management, most patients can achieve some degree of pain-free motion. Treatment should be focused on symptom management and prevention of progression.

Therapeutic Modalities

Splinting, either with a custom design or over-the-counter thumb splint at night or on a wearing schedule can result in reasonable pain relief. This can be of particular benefit during acute flares.

Strengthening exercises and joint ROM can help desensitize the joint's innervating nerves, allowing for increased use while decreasing sensitivity to pain. Use of hot and cold packs can help alleviate pain, or aid in muscle relaxation before completing aggravating tasks.

Pharmacological Management

NSAIDs, either topical or oral, may be utilized to address pain and decrease swelling.

Interventional Medicine

For moderate disease, corticosteroid injections can be beneficial for pain relief. However, repetitive injections may lead to joint weakening. Hyaluronic acid injections have shown no relief in pain or improved functioning when compared to corticosteroids [33].

Surgery is an option for end-stage cases refractory to conservative care [34].

2.2.7 Radial Sensory Neuritis

Wartenberg syndrome, Handcuff neuropathy, cheiralgia paresthetica

2.2.7.1 Overview
Irritation of the radial sensory nerve can occur alone, or in conjunction with radial styloid tenosynovitis. As a purely sensory nerve, this syndrome presents without motor symptoms.

2.2.7.2 Pathogenesis
The superficial branch of the radial nerve (RSN) arises in the proximal forearm from the bifurcation of the radial nerve. It then courses deep to the brachioradialis, travelling through the deep fascia, and emerges around 10 cm proximal to the radial styloid between the brachioradialis and ECRL in the dorsal compartment. Near its terminal end, it courses close to the skin. The nerve itself then bifurcates, with the dorsal branch supplying sensory innervation to the first and second web space and palmar branch supplying sensory innervation to the dorsolateral thumb.

The sensory distribution is shared with the median nerve and dorsal ulnar cutaneous nerve. This is clinically important as a pure sensory deficit might be difficult to localize.

The nerve can be compressed either internally or externally. During repetitive wrist and thumb movements, the sensory radial nerve can become compressed between the brachioradialis and ECRL tendons. Similarly, wristwatches, bracelets, or compression gloves may serve as an extrinsic cause of injury. With the advent of nonscientifically backed performance gloves in the esports sphere, this syndrome is of particular clinical importance [35].

2.2.7.3 Presentation

Patients may complain of radiating pain as well as sensory deficits, paresthesias, and dysesthesia across the thumb and dorsoradial hand. Pain is often ill-defined and poorly localized. Symptoms often worsen with wrist flexion and ulnar deviation. Patients may also state they no longer wear bracelets and wristwatches as a result. For teams with long-sleeved jerseys, clinicians may pick up on competitors rolling up one sleeve over the other [36].

> **Clinical Pearl**
> RSN can be associated with radial styloid tenosynovitis in up to half of cases [37].

2.2.7.4 Diagnosis

As the radial sensory nerve is purely sensory, any motor involvement that is found on physical exam should point to another, more proximal etiology.

Physical Examination

Sensory examination will reveal decreased or abnormal sensation in the dorsal thumb and dorsal radial hand. Given the overlapping dermatomes of the hand, the dorsal web space of the thumb can be most precise to localize purely RSN lesions.

If the cause is secondary to concurrent radial styloid tenosynovitis, then Finkelstein's test may also be performed.

> **Clinical Pearl**
> Radial Sensory Neuritis Versus
>
> - Radial Styloid Tenosynovitis. RSN is often aggravated by pronation, where tenosynovitis is aggravated by ulnar deviation.
> - Intersection syndrome: RSN will not present with crepitus with wrist flexion/extension.

Tinel's Test
There may be a positive Tinel's sign over the radial sensory nerve.

Hyperpronation Provocative Testing
With the wrist held in ulnar deviation, the forearm is pronated. Paresthesias in the distribution of the RSN signifies a positive test.

Imaging
Imaging and electrodiagnostics are of little use. When the diagnosis is unclear, a diagnostic wrist block of the RSN can be performed. The test would be considered positive if it provides temporary symptomatic relief.

Electrodiagnostics
Patients with purely radial sensory neuritis may have abnormal sensory nerve conduction values on NCS. They should have otherwise normal NCS and EMGs, and abnormality would point in the direction of an alternative diagnosis [38].

2.2.7.5 Treatment
Given that the nerve is purely sensory, numbness is the only clinical consequence of lack of treatment. As such, options that offer more complicated risks should be avoided. If the neuritis arises secondary to radial styloid tenosynovitis, treatment of the causative factor should take precedent.

Therapeutic Modalities
A thumb spica splint may alleviate painful dysesthesia. However, a splint that is too tight may worsen symptoms. Patients should be instructed to avoid tight clothing and watches.

Implementing a routine, including radial and median nerve glides, not to exceed more than 10 individual glides a day, can help prevent RSN. These exercises reinforce the proper pathway for the nerve and other structures to decrease the risk of entrapment or compression [36].

2.3   Elbow

2.3.1   Ulnar Neuropathy

Cubital Tunnel Syndrome, Guyon's Canal Syndrome, Funny
Bone

2.3.1.1 Overview
The ulnar nerve is the largest unprotected nerve in the human
body, leaving it susceptible to damage in a multitude of places.
Ulnar neuropathy can occur both at the wrist and the elbow, with
the latter being far more common, and is the second most common compression neuropathy. The ulnar nerve provides motor
innervation to part of the forearm and majority of the hand, as
well as sensory innervation to the hand.

2.3.1.2 Pathogenesis
As the ulnar nerve courses from its origin at the medial cord of the
brachial plexus to its terminal destination, there are a multitude of
possible places for entrapment or compression. In the upper arm,
the ulnar nerve pierces the Arcade of Struthers, a musculoaponeu-
rotic canal and site of potential pathology. It then travels distally
along the humerus and enters the retrocondylar groove, also
known as the cubital tunnel. The tunnel is bound by the flexor
carpi ulnaris muscle, humeroulnar arcade, and medial elbow ligaments. This site is the most common area of compression, due in
part to its dynamic size with elbow movement. Of note, some
authors choose to separate the retrocondylar groove from the
cubital tunnel. However, for the scope of this book, they will be
discussed as a similar structure.

With elbow flexion, the space between the medial epicondyle and olecranon increases by up to 1 cm. Subsequently, the
humeroulnar arcade tightens down upon the ulnar nerve. At the
same time, the medial elbow ligaments bulge and flatten the
floor of the normally deep retrocondylar groove, while the
medial head of the triceps muscle pushes the nerve posteriorly.
When the elbow is in complete flexion, the nerve is pulled tight
around the medial epicondyle. This is a significantly different

orientation from extension, during which the ulnar nerve is freely movable.

Compression or damage at this site is labeled cubital tunnel syndrome. In the esports population, this is usually a result of chronic mechanical compression from arm rests and desks or stretch from chronic elbow flexion. It can also result from a fracture of the medial epicondyle of the humerus (causing direct ulnar nerve injury) or fracture of the lateral epicondyle of the humerus, which may result in a valgus deformity at the elbow.

The nerve then pierces the aponeurosis lining the deep heads of the flexor carpi ulnaris and runs between the tendons and muscle planes of the medial forearm to the wrist.

In the mid-forearm, two sensory branches arise from the ulnar nerve, the palmar cutaneous branch and dorsal cutaneous branch, and course distally, avoiding the Guyon canal. The former supplies the cutaneous territory over the proximal border of the ulnar portion of the palm. The latter supplies the ulnar side of the dorsum of the hand and dorsal surfaces of the fifth and ulnar half of the fourth digit.

The ulnar nerve enters the hand via Guyon's canal, along with the ulnar artery, which is bound superficially by the flexor retinaculum and medially by the pisiform bone. As the nerve exits the groove, it passes under the aponeurotic arch of the humeroulnar arcade (a derivative of the flexor carpi ulnaris muscle). The roof of Guyon's canal consists of the palmar fascia and the palmaris brevis muscle. The nerve may also be compressed at this location, either directly from the surface of a desk or a Guyon's canal cyst.

The ulnar nerve provides sensory innervation to the fifth digit and medial half of the fourth digit, as well as dorsal medial hand and medial forearm. It also provides motor innervation to a number of forearm and hand muscles, most relevantly the forearm flexors, including the muscles of the hypothenar eminence [39].

2.3.1.3 Presentation

Sensory and motor complaints distal to the site of compression are the hallmarks of ulnar nerve damage. Numbness or paresthesia in the medial forearm that radiates into the pinkie and ring finger are common complaints. Patients may not initially be able to localize the specific involved digits initially, but are often more successful when more targeted questions are presented.

Sensory changes can be localized over the hypothenar eminence, as well as the ulnar half of the palm, fifth and medial half of the fourth digit. These can manifest as paresthesia and numbness. Patients may also complain of pain, which is more commonly around the elbow. Symptoms are often worse at night or with repetitive elbow/wrist movements.

Motor weakness present can be subclinical. Patients with severe compression or transection can complain of weakness in wrist flexion or be unable to cross their fingers. Weakness of the pinkie finger may result in difficulty placing the little finger into their pocket.

Ulnar lesions at the elbow typically present with numbness and tingling in the fourth and fifth digits, medial elbow pain, nocturnal numbness and paresthesia, and worsening of symptoms with elbow and/or repeated wrist flexion. Ulnar lesions at the wrist typically present with hand weakness and atrophy, loss of dexterity, and variable sensory involvement as outlined below.

Sensory symptoms from ulnar neuropathy at the elbow are often brought on by sustained elbow flexion (e.g., when talking on the phone or lying on one's side with the elbow flexed). Symptoms can also be provoked by leaning on the elbow or when performing activity that requires sustained or repetitive grip, or repeated forearm pronation and supination). Patients may complain of weakness and clumsiness of the hands, most specifically in activities that require hand dexterity, such as their keyboard hand or when buttoning [40].

Clinical Pearl
Loss of dexterity due to ulnar neuropathy is usually indicative of weakness of the intrinsic hand muscles in contrast to mild median nerve injury, where loss of dexterity is most often related to sensory loss.

2.3.1.4 Diagnosis

The diagnosis of ulnar neuropathy at the elbow or wrist can be made clinically via effective history taking and a thorough physical examination. If the clinical picture is uncertain, electrodiagnostics and imaging may be necessary.

Physical Examination

Inspection can reveal interossei and hypothenar eminence atrophy. Some degree of thenar eminence atrophy may also be present, secondary to wasting of the ulnar-innervated adductor pollicis and deep head of the flexor pollicis brevis. With long-standing damage, a claw hand deformity, also known as Benediction posture, can develop at rest. This results from hyperextension of the 4th and 5th digits and the metacarpophalangeal joints and flexion of the interphalangeal joints. This is more common with injuries at the wrist as opposed to the upper arm, as the ulnar half of the flexor digitorum profundus is spare, pulling the DIP joints into a more flexed position (also known as ulnar paradox). Inspection may also reveal Wartenberg's sign, which is the little finger held into abduction secondary to weakness.

The ulnar nerve can be palpated in the elbow region, with special attention being paid for any swelling or masses. Subluxation can be assessed over the medial epicondyle, while flexing and extending at the elbow. Examiners may feel a snapping sensation.

A sensory examination may reveal diminished sensation over the aforementioned regions, and splitting of the fourth digit. Injury to the ulnar nerve at the wrist can produce remarkably different clinical pictures depending on the area of damage. Injury to the ulnar nerve, before it divides into smaller tributaries in Guyon's canal, will have broader sensory consequences and affect all ulnar innervated intrinsic hand muscles. Distal to Guyon's canal, injuries to the deep terminal motor branch and superficial terminal branch will have varying clinical consequences, outside the scope of this textbook.

Tinel's Test

To perform, sustained, light percussion is applied to the ulnar nerve at the elbow or wrist. Paresthesias along the distribution of the nerve is considered a positive test.

Froment's Sign

The patient is instructed to pinch a sheet of paper between their thumb and pointer finger while holding the thumb IP joint in extension. Patients with ulnar nerve damage and subsequent weakness of the adductor pollicis will flex their fingers in order to maintain grip strength, thus compensating with their median-nerve innervated flexor pollicis longus. Patients with a positive Fromen's sign will be unable to hold the extended thumb posture, as shown in Fig. 2.8.

Imaging

Advanced imaging is useful when the clinical picture is murky, and may be particularly helpful when masses (such as ganglion cysts) are present.

Ultrasound examination may reveal altered echogenicity, enlargement and entrapment of the nerve, and transposition. Enlargement of the nerve proximal to the site of entrapment is a common finding. After the ulnar nerve is localized at the elbow, the arm can be flexed and extended to assess for possible subluxation.

One study suggests that sonographic evaluation of ulnar neuropathy of the elbow based upon nerve diameter may have a sensitivity and specificity of 80 and 91% compared to clinical and electrodiagnostic criteria alone. When compared to electrodiagnostic diagnosis, another study showed a sensitivity and specificity of 95% and 71%.

MRI may reveal increased signal intensity on T2-weighted or STIR imaging sequences as well as increased size of the ulnar nerve [41, 42].

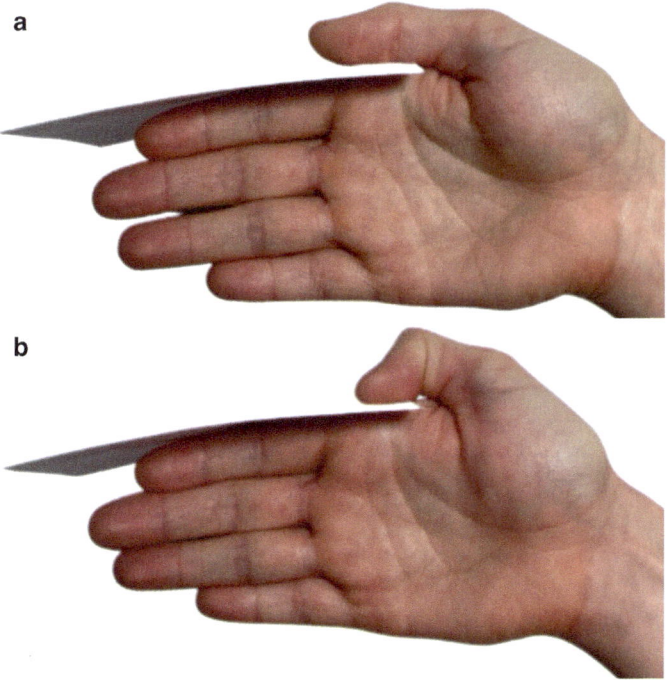

Fig. 2.8 (**a**) Normal thumb adduction (**b**) Positive Froment's sign, as signified by flexion of the thumb's interphalangeal joint

Electrodiagnostics

Nerve conduction studies are relatively straightforward in the evaluation of ulnar neuropathy. Abnormalities may be found when testing ulnar sensory responses to the fifth digit, or when testing motor studies are recorded to the abductor digiti minimi. For equivocal results around the elbow, an "inching" technique can be applied, also known as short segment incremental studies. This can be helpful in locating the exact location of the lesion.

Furthermore, dual channel studies may be done by recording over the ADM and first dorsal interosseous (FDI) simultaneously. The FDI destined nerve fibers run more peripherally across the elbow, placing them at a higher risk for compression.

2.3.1.5 Treatment

Therapeutic Modalities
If the inciting trauma is found to be extrinsic compression from position while gaming, elbow pads can aid in both prevention of aggravation and treatment. Pads are placed on the dorsal-medial elbow during waking hours to prevent compression over the medial epicondyle. This can then be rotated to the ante-cubital fossa at night, thereby preventing excessive flexion. A simple towel can also be utilized during sleep hours to the same effect. Activity modification is equally as important for ulnar neuropathy at the wrist. Padded gloves may be utilized, or a wrist rest that avoids direct compression to Guyon's canal.

Referral to an occupational therapist may also include incorporation of nerve gliding exercises as well as soft tissue release of the forearm [43].

Pharmacological Management
The role of pharmacological management is limited in ulnar neuropathy. Oral NSAIDs may be helpful in acute phases for pain control.

Interventional Medicine
In severe cases, the nerve may need to be surgically released from its area of entrapment. Surgery is often indicated for patients with clear weakness, sensory loss, or signs of denervation on EMG. Surgery of the elbow usually includes simple decompression by cutting the humeroulnar arcade (flexor carpi ulnaris aponeurosis) or transposition. The latter is performed by first cutting the aponeurosis and then mobilizing the ulnar nerve anteriorly from the retrocondylar groove. In severe cases, a medial epicondylectomy may be performed.

Most of the available data for ulnar neuropathy at the elbow suggest that ulnar nerve decompression and transposition result in similar clinical outcomes, though transposition may be hampered by higher rates of complications. On top of lower rates of complications, decompression procedures are faster and less technically demanding [44, 45].

2.3.2 Lateral Epicondylitis

Tennis elbow, elbow tendinopathy, lateral epicondylalgia, elbow tendonitis

2.3.2.1 Overview
The lateral epicondyle of the elbow is the bony origin for the majority of the wrist extensors. Pain at the myotendinous junction of these muscle groups is referred to as lateral epicondylitis. This diagnosis was initially described in 1883 associated with lawn tennis, but this chronic tendinosis is of increasing concern in the gaming population due to its association with repetitive or dysfunction wrist extension.

2.3.2.2 Pathogenesis
The lateral epicondyle is an extra-articular bony prominence on the distal humerus that serves as the common origin of the wrist extensors. The most common involved muscle is the extensor carpi radialis brevis muscle (ECRB) followed by the extensor digitorum communis muscle (EDC). Involvement of the extensor carpi radialis longus or extensor carpi ulnaris is rare.

Despite the -itis suffix, histological examination of epicondylitis reveals very few inflammatory cells. Evidence suggests that epicondylitis is not an acute inflammatory reaction, but rather a result of chronic tendinosis. Eccentric movement, referring to any movement that lengthens a muscle at the same time it is being contracted, is the most common indicated mechanism of injury. Chronic, repetitive eccentric motion can lead to disorganized tissue structure, placing the muscle at further risk for injury [46].

2.3.2.3 Presentation
Pain in the lateral elbow is the most common presenting symptom, often exacerbated by wrist and elbow movement as well as radial deviation. Patients with epicondylitis typically complain of extra-articular elbow pain. The pain's severity can range from having a minimal effect on sports or work activities to severely impairing basic daily tasks and sleep.

Symptom onset is traditionally gradual, with aggravating after specific activities that involve gripping and wrist extension. Players may complain of pain in either their keyboard or controller hands, and it may worsen when reaching thumb-sided keybinds. Symptoms are worsened after long gaming sessions that do not involve scheduled breaks.

2.3.2.4 Diagnosis

Physical Examination
Palpation can elicit pain at the lateral epicondyle and immediate wrist extensor muscle mass. The ECRB can be palpated just at the tip of the lateral epicondyle, and the EDC posterior and distal to that.

Range of motion testing can reveal pain with passive wrist flexion to end range. Resisted wrist extension, third digit extension, pronation, and supination may also cause discomfort.

Cozen's Test
The patient's arm is placed in a position of complete elbow extension and forearm pronation with a clenched fist. The examiner stabilizes the elbow with one hand while palpating the lateral epicondyle, and the other hand is placed on the dorsum of the patient's hand. The patient then extends and radially deviates the wrist. Pain over the lateral epicondyle represents a positive test.

> **Clinical Pearl**
> The fingers are flexed in a fist to avoid involvement of the extensor digitorium origin. Similarly, radial counterforce is also applied by the examiner to avoid involvement of the extensor carpi ulnaris and confounding by concurrent ECU tendonitis.

Imaging

Imaging should be reserved for cases refractory to conservative management, and is not necessary for straightforward diagnoses. Three-view x-ray series may reveal underlying bony abnormalities, such as long-standing osteoarthritic changes or heterotopic ossification.

Musculoskeletal ultrasound can identify abnormal tendon appearance (e.g., tendon thickening, partial tear at tendon origin, calcifications). MRI may reveal increased signal intensity on T2 weighted images in ECRB [47].

2.3.2.5 Treatment

Therapeutic Modalities

Activity modification, counterforce bracing, NSAIDs, and physical therapy are the mainstays of treatment. Without intervention, epicondylitis can take upwards of two years to resolve.

Counterforce bracing may provide benefit in acute flares by reducing the stress on the muscular insertion point. This circular brace is placed approximately 6–10 cm distal to the elbow joint. Studies conducted by independent researchers and not manufacturer-supported are scant, but bracing may reduce pain and, therefore, contribute to functionality. Splinting with a volar wrist splint is of little use and has not been found to be more effective than a counterforce brace, but is significantly more cumbersome. Splinting may also be associated with poorer outcomes.

Physical and occupational therapy focused on progressive eccentric strengthening may also be effective. Both the extensor and supinator groups should be targeted. Common utilized exercises include utilizing wrist flexion with resistance band, going from complete extension to complete flexion. Gamers should be encouraged to warm up prior to play, focusing on range of motion exercises, as well as self-massage their forearm muscles to reduce stiffness [48–50].

Pharmacological Management

Oral NSAIDs may be indicated in the short term to reduce pain and improve function, but caution must be taken for long-term usage given the propensity of side effects. Topical NSAIDs may provide some symptomatic relief given the superficial nature of the indicated structures.

Interventional Medicine

If standard interventions prove unsuccessful, more aggressive interventions can be pursued. However, if imaging has not yet been obtained, further diagnostics may be indicated.

Corticosteroid injections have been shown to lead to worse long-term outcomes and do not prevent recurrences, and should be considered in cases where immediate pain relief is the primary concern. While short-term pain relief may be better when compared to no injection, it has been associated with a higher rate of recurrence [50, 51].

"Peppering," a technique in which the tendon is injected upwards of 50 times, is an interesting approach that has been shown to lead to better outcomes than placebo. Results found were independent of medication administered, suggesting the effect is related to the injection technique rather than the injectable. This intervention may be deemed beneficial via an invoked inflammatory response, similar to PRP injections discussed later [52].

As mentioned previously, lateral epicondylitis is a chronic condition resulting in disorganized tissue architecture. A growing field of treatment, known as "proinflammatory" has been proposed to reverse these chronic changes by stimulating the inflammatory response. These interventions are still in their infancy, and as a result, lack high-quality research studies. Platelet-rich plasma injections thought to be rich in growth factors that will theoretically stimulate tissue repair have been utilized by regenerative medicine proponents [53].

Other interventions have been proposed and have varying degrees of efficacy. There is no evidence that extracorporeal shock wave therapy or acupuncture produce long-term benefits. Studies addressing the use of botulinum toxin A at the myotendinous junction have shown a reduction in symptoms without decreases in grip strength. Prolotherapy, injecting an irritant, such as dextrose, in an effort to simulate a local inflammatory response, has also been utilized [54, 55].

2.3.3 Olecranon Bursitis

2.3.3.1 Overview
The olecranon bursa is a fluid-filled sac overlying the posterior elbow designed to reduce joint friction. Inflammation of that sac can occur with longstanding microtrauma, such as leaning on the elbow, resulting in painless swelling. Of minimal clinical significance, this pathology will be discussed briefly.

2.3.3.2 Pathogenesis
Normal bursa are essentially empty sacs, with almost no, or only a small amount of fluid present. Under physiological conditions, the bursa serves to reduce joint friction. In pathological states, the bursa becomes inflamed, subsequently increasing fluid production. Increased fluid causes the cavity to swell, ballooning out.

Bursitis most commonly develops from trauma. One single injury to the elbow is more common in the general population. In the gaming population, a buildup of microtraumas from constant pressure on the olecranon during gaming is a more common etiology.

2.3.3.3 Presentation
Patients will commonly present with swelling over the posterior olecranon process. This is most often painless swelling, but can present with pain or redness.

2.3.3.4 Diagnosis

Physical Examination
The bursa is located over the proximal end of the ulna on the extensor aspect. Normal, non-inflamed bursa are usually not able

to be palpated. A palpable bursa is the most obvious sign of bursitis.

The olecranon bursa is an extra-articular structure; therefore, the fluid buildup is not in the joint. As a result, range of motion will not be affected. Superficial skin lesions may indicate infection of the bursa, a condition that may warrant fluid aspiration and testing.

Imaging
A thorough physical examination should be the only necessary diagnostic step.

2.3.3.5 Treatment

Therapeutic Modalities
Prevention of further microtraumas should be the mainstay. An evaluation of a player's setup may be necessary if the bursitis does not resolve quickly. PC gamers should be encouraged to rest their forearms on their desk, rather than the elbows directly. Console gamers may similarly be assuming a more acute elbow flexion angle, thus placing increased pressure on the bursa. Education and prevention may fully resolve the swelling. If further intervention is necessary, compression may help reduce inflammation and encourage fluid reduction [55].

References

1. Nagle DJ. Evaluation of chronic wrist pain. J Am Acad Orthop Surg. 2000;8(1):45–55. https://doi.org/10.5435/00124635-200001000-00005.
2. Ihnatsenka B, Boezaart AP. Ultrasound: basic understanding and learning the language. Int J Shoulder Surg. 2010;4(3):55–62. https://doi.org/10.4103/0973-6042.76960.
3. Zlatkin MB, Chao PC, Osterman AL, Schnall MD, Dalinka MK, Kressel HY. Chronic wrist pain: evaluation with high-resolution MR imaging. Radiology. 1989;173(3):723–9. https://doi.org/10.1148/radiology.173.3.2813777.
4. Tavee J. Nerve conduction studies: basic concepts. Handb Clin Neurol. 2019;160:217–24. https://doi.org/10.1016/B978-0-444-64032-1.00014-X.

5. Preston D, Shapiro B. Electromyography and neuromuscular disorders E-book. 3rd ed. London: Saunders; 2012.
6. Malanga GA, Yan N, Stark J. Mechanisms and efficacy of heat and cold therapies for musculoskeletal injury. Postgrad Med. 2015;127(1):57–65. https://doi.org/10.1080/00325481.2015.992719.
7. Parreira Pdo C, Costa Lda C, Hespanhol LC Jr, Lopes AD, Costa LO. Current evidence does not support the use of Kinesio taping in clinical practice: a systematic review. J Physiother. 2014;60(1):31–9. https://doi.org/10.1016/j.jphys.2013.12.008.
8. Eraslan L, Yuce D, Erbilici A, Baltaci G. Does Kinesiotaping improve pain and functionality in patients with newly diagnosed lateral epicondylitis? Knee Surg Sports Traumatol Arthrosc. 2018;26(3):938–45. https://doi.org/10.1007/s00167-017-4691-7.
9. Wiffen PJ, Derry S, Moore RA, Aldington D, Cole P, Rice ASC, et al. Antiepileptic drugs for neuropathic pain and fibromyalgia – an overview of cochrane reviews. Cochrane Database Syst Rev. 2013;11:CD010567. https://doi.org/10.1002/14651858.CD010567.pub2.
10. Roy AJ, Roy AN, De C, Banerji D, Das S, Chatterjee B, et al. A cadaveric study of the first dorsal compartment of the wrist and its content tendons: anatomical variations in the Indian population. J Hand Microsurg. 2012;4(2):55–9. https://doi.org/10.1007/s12593-012-0073-z.
11. Clarke MT, Lyall HA, Grant JW, Matthewson MH. The histopathology of de Quervain's disease. J Hand Surg Br. 1998;23(6):732–4. https://doi.org/10.1016/s0266-7681(98)80085-5.
12. Ippolito E, Postacchini F, Scola E, Bellocci M, De Martino C. De Quervain's disease. An ultrastructural study. Int Orthop. 1985;9(1):41–7. https://doi.org/10.1007/BF00267036.
13. Ashraf MO, Devadoss VG. Systematic review and meta-analysis on steroid injection therapy for de Quervain's tenosynovitis in adults. Eur J Orthop Surg Traumatol. 2014;24(2):149–57. https://doi.org/10.1007/s00590-012-1164-z.
14. Scheller A, Schuh R, Hönle W, Schuh A. Long-term results of surgical release of de Quervain's stenosing tenosynovitis. Int Orthop. 2009;33(5):1301–3. https://doi.org/10.1007/s00264-008-0667-z.
15. Hoy G, Trease L, Braybon W. Intersection syndrome: an acute surgical disease in elite rowers. BMJ Open Sport Exerc Med. 2019;5(1):e000535. https://doi.org/10.1136/bmjsem-2019-000535.
16. Giovagnorio F, Miozzi F. Ultrasound findings in intersection syndrome. J Med Ultrason. 2012;39(4):217–20. https://doi.org/10.1007/s10396-012-0370-y.
17. Hanlon DP, Luellen JR. Intersection syndrome: a case report and review of the literature. J Emerg Med. 1999;17(6):969–71. https://doi.org/10.1016/s0736-4679(99)00125-0.
18. Campbell D, Campbell R, O'Connor P, Hawkes R. Sports-related extensor carpi ulnaris pathology: a review of functional anatomy, sports injury

and management. Br J Sports Med. 2013;47(17):1105–11. https://doi.org/10.1136/bjsports-2013-092835.

19. Montalvan B, Parier J, Brasseur JL, Le Viet D, Drape JL. Extensor carpi ulnaris injuries in tennis players: a study of 28 cases. Br J Sports Med. 2006;40(5):424–9. https://doi.org/10.1136/bjsm.2005.023275.

20. Ruland RT, Hogan CJ. The ECU synergy test: an aid to diagnose ECU tendonitis. J Hand Surg Am. 2008;33(10):1777–82. https://doi.org/10.1016/j.jhsa.2008.08.018.

21. Simoneau GG, Marklin RW, Berman JE. Effect of computer keyboard slope on wrist position and forearm electromyography of typists without musculoskeletal disorders. Phys Ther. 2003;83(9):816–30.

22. Spinner M, Kaplan EB. Extensor carpi ulnaris. Its relationship to the stability of the distal radio-ulnar joint. Clin Orthop Relat Res. 1970;68:124–9.

23. Seradge H, Jia YC, Owens W. In vivo measurement of carpal tunnel pressure in the functioning hand. J Hand Surg Am. 1995;20(5):855–9. https://doi.org/10.1016/S0363-5023(05)80443-5.

24. Szabo RM, Chidgey LK. Stress carpal tunnel pressures in patients with carpal tunnel syndrome and normal patients. J Hand Surg Am. 1989;14(4):624–7. https://doi.org/10.1016/0363-5023(89)90178-0.

25. Bland JD. A neurophysiological grading scale for carpal tunnel syndrome. Muscle Nerve. 2000;23(8):1280–3. https://doi.org/10.1002/1097-4598(200008)23:8<1280::aid-mus20>3.0.co;2-y.

26. Bland JD. Do nerve conduction studies predict the outcome of carpal tunnel decompression? Muscle Nerve. 2001;24(7):935–40. https://doi.org/10.1002/mus.1091.

27. Kleinman WB. Stability of the distal radioulna joint: biomechanics, pathophysiology, physical diagnosis, and restoration of function what we have learned in 25 years. J Hand Surg Am. 2007;32(7):1086–106. https://doi.org/10.1016/j.jhsa.2007.06.014.

28. Ahn AK, Chang D, Plate AM. Triangular fibrocartilage complex tears: a review. Bull NYU Hosp Jt Dis. 2006;64(3–4):114–8.

29. Prosser R, Harvey L, Lastayo P, Hargreaves I, Scougall P, Herbert RD. Provocative wrist tests and MRI are of limited diagnostic value for suspected wrist ligament injuries: a cross-sectional study. J Physiother. 2011;57(4):247–53. https://doi.org/10.1016/S1836-9553(11)70055-8.

30. Barlow SJ. A non-surgical intervention for triangular fibrocartilage complex tears. Physiother Res Int. 2016;21(4):271–6. https://doi.org/10.1002/pri.1672.

31. Shih JT, Hou YT, Lee HM, Tan CM. Chronic triangular fibrocartilage complex tears with distal radioulna joint instability: a new method of triangular fibrocartilage complex reconstruction. J Orthop Surg (Hong Kong). 2000;8(1):1–8. https://doi.org/10.1177/230949900000800102.

32. Peter JB, Marmor L. Osteoarthritis of the first carpometacarpal joint. Calif Med. 1968;109(2):116–20.

33. Kroon FP, Rubio R, Schoones JW, Kloppenburg M. Intra-articular thera-
    pies in the treatment of hand osteoarthritis: a systematic literature review.
    Drugs Aging. 2016;33(2):119–33. https://doi.org/10.1007/s40266-015-
    0330-5.
34. Ghavami A, Oishi SN. Thumb trapeziometacarpal arthritis: treatment
    with ligament reconstruction tendon interposition arthroplasty. Plast
    Reconstr Surg. 2006;117(6):116e–28e. https://doi.org/10.1097/01.
    prs.0000214652.31293.23.
35. Han BR, Cho YJ, Yang JS, Kang SH, Choi HJ. Clinical features of wrist
    drop caused by compressive radial neuropathy and its anatomical
    considerations. J Korean Neurosurg Soc. 2014;55(3):148–51. https://doi.
    org/10.3340/jkns.2014.55.3.148.
36. Wang LH, Weiss MD. Anatomical, clinical, and electrodiagnostic fea-
    tures of radial neuropathies. Phys Med Rehabil Clin N Am. 2013;24(1):33–
    47. https://doi.org/10.1016/j.pmr.2012.08.018.
37. Lanzetta M, Foucher G. Entrapment of the superficial branch of the radial
    nerve (Wartenberg's syndrome). A report of 52 cases. Int Orthop.
    1993;17(6):342–5. https://doi.org/10.1007/BF00180450.
38. Frontera WR. Cyclist's palsy: clinical and electrodiagnostic findings. Br
    J Sports Med. 1983;17(2):91–3. https://doi.org/10.1136/bjsm.17.2.91.
39. Padua L, Aprile I, Caliandro P, Foschini M, Mazza S, Tonali P. Natural
    history of ulnar entrapment at elbow. Clin Neurophysiol.
    2002;113(12):1980–4. https://doi.org/10.1016/s1388-2457(02)00295-x.
40. Frost P, Johnsen B, Fuglsang-Frederiksen A, Svendsen SW. Lifestyle risk
    factors for ulnar neuropathy and ulnar neuropathy-like symptoms. Muscle
    Nerve. 2013;48(4):507–15. https://doi.org/10.1002/mus.23820.
41. Bayrak AO, Bayrak IK, Turker H, Elmali M, Nural MS. Ultrasonography
    in patients with ulnar neuropathy at the elbow: comparison of cross-
    sectional area and swelling ratio with electrophysiological severity.
    Muscle Nerve. 2010;41(5):661–6. https://doi.org/10.1002/mus.21563.
42. Beekman R, Schoemaker MC, Van Der Plas JP, et al. Diagnostic value
    of high-resolution sonography in ulnar neuropathy at the elbow.
    Neurology. 2004;62(5):767–73. https://doi.org/10.1212/01.wnl.000011
    3733.62689.0d.
43. Caliandro P, La Torre G, Padua R, Giannini F, Padua L. Treatment for
    ulnar neuropathy at the elbow. Cochrane Database Syst Rev.
    2016;11(11):CD006839. https://doi.org/10.1002/14651858.CD006839.
    pub4.
44. Brown JM, Yee A, Mackinnon SE. Distal median to ulnar nerve transfers
    to restore ulnar motor and sensory function within the hand: technical
    nuances. Neurosurgery. 2009;65(5):966–78. https://doi.org/10.1227/01.
    NEU.0000358951.64043.73.
45. Davidge KM, Yee A, Moore AM, Mackinnon SE. The supercharge end-
    to-side anterior interosseous-to-ulnar motor nerve transfer for restoring

intrinsic function: clinical experience. Plast Reconstr Surg. 2015;136(3):344e–52e.https://doi.org/10.1097/PRS.0000000000001514.
46. Cohen M, da Rocha Motta Filho G. Lateral epicondylitis of the elbow. Rev Bras Ortop. 2015;47(4):414–20. https://doi.org/10.1016/S2255-4971(15)30121-X.
47. Chen AL, Youm T, Ong BC, Rafii M, Rokito AS. Imaging of the elbow in the overhead throwing athlete. Am J Sports Med. 2003;31(3):466–73. https://doi.org/10.1177/03635465030310032601.
48. Hoogvliet P, Randsdorp MS, Dingemanse R, Koes BW, Huisstede BM. Does effectiveness of exercise therapy and mobilisation techniques offer guidance for the treatment of lateral and medial epicondylitis? A systematic review. Br J Sports Med. 2013;47(17):1112–9. https://doi.org/10.1136/bjsports-2012-091990.
49. Van De Streek MD, Van Der Schans CP, De Greef MH, Postema K. The effect of a forearm/hand splint compared with an elbow band as a treatment for lateral epicondylitis. Prosthetics Orthot Int. 2004;28(2):183–9. https://doi.org/10.1080/03093640408726703.
50. Croisier JL, Foidart-Dessalle M, Tinant F, Crielaard JM, Forthomme B. An isokinetic eccentric programme for the management of chronic lateral epicondylar tendinopathy. Br J Sports Med. 2007;41(4):269–75. https://doi.org/10.1136/bjsm.2006.033324.
51. Olaussen M, Holmedal O, Lindbaek M, Brage S, Solvang H. Treating lateral epicondylitis with corticosteroid injections or non-electrotherapeutical physiotherapy: a systematic review. BMJ Open. 2013;3(10):e003564. https://doi.org/10.1136/bmjopen-2013-003564.
52. Mishra AK, Skrepnik NV, Edwards SG, et al. Efficacy of platelet-rich plasma for chronic tennis elbow: a double-blind, prospective, multicenter, randomized controlled trial of 230 patients. Am J Sports Med. 2014;42(2):463–71. https://doi.org/10.1177/0363546513494359.
53. Espandar R, Heidari P, Rasouli MR, et al. Use of anatomic measurement to guide injection of botulinum toxin for the management of chronic lateral epicondylitis: a randomized controlled trial. CMAJ. 2010;182(8):768–73. https://doi.org/10.1503/cmaj.090906.
54. Scarpone M, Rabago DP, Zgierska A, Arbogast G, Snell E. The efficacy of prolotherapy for lateral epicondylosis: a pilot study. Clin J Sport Med. 2008;18(3):248–54. https://doi.org/10.1097/JSM.0b013e318170fc87.
55. Reilly D, Kamineni S. Olecranon bursitis. J Shoulder Elb Surg. 2016;25(1):158–67. https://doi.org/10.1016/j.jse.2015.08.032.

Neck and Back Disorders in Esports

3

Lindsey Migliore and Caitlin McGee

3.1 Overview

Nonspecific, also known as mechanical, back pain is one of the most frequently encountered medical conditions and will be experienced by >85% of people during the course of their lifetime. As with any other joint of the body, the spine gradually degenerates with age. However, due to poor posture and ergonomic negligence, the gaming population may be at higher risk for early degeneration.

While the source of pain in this population may commonly be the mundane and benign myofascial origin that requires no advanced imaging or interventions, it still requires aggressive provider involvement. Focus should be paid on ergonomic interventions, informed counselling, and tailored exercise programs to prevent acute processes from advancing into chronic [1].

In a case study of college esports athletes, 42% of players experienced neck or back pain [2]. Extended desk times, poor

L. Migliore (✉)
GamerDoc, Washington, DC, USA
e-mail: doc@gamerdoc.net

C. McGee
1HP, Washington, DC, USA

© The Author(s), under exclusive license to Springer Nature Switzerland AG 2021
L. Migliore et al. (eds.), *Handbook of Esports Medicine*,
https://doi.org/10.1007/978-3-030-73610-1_3

posture, core weakness, and inactivity can compound and predispose patients to a multitude of degenerative changes.

Because the field of esports medicine is in its infancy, practitioners must rely on their knowledge of anatomy and pathophysiology when the precedent fails them and research studies are absent.

3.1.1 Anatomy

The vertebral column is a major component of the axial skeleton composed of 24 bony vertebrae separated by intervertebral discs. Vertebrae are named according to their spinal region, with 7 cervical, 12 thoracic, 5 lumbar, 5 fused sacral, and 4 fused coccyx components. Each vertebrae contains structures intended for joint articulation and muscle attachments, as well as openings, called foramina, for spinal nerve roots. The vertebrae are anatomically divided into two parts: the anterior vertebral body and posterior vertebral arch.

The posterior vertebral arch houses and protects the spinal cord, and is formed by two pedicles, two laminae, and seven processes (one spinous, two transverse, and four articular). Facet joints, also known as zygapophyseal or apophyseal joints, are true synovial joints formed between the articular processes of two adjacent vertebrae. Each facet joint contains a capsule, meniscus, and synovial membrane. Facet joints, shown in Fig. 3.1, guide movement of their corresponding spinal segment and provide stabilization.

The facet joint has nociceptive receptors in both the capsule and synovium. Each joint receives dual innervation from medial branches of the dorsal primary ramus of the corresponding spinal nerve. Facet joints in the cervical spine are innervated by the same level, and the level below, whereas those in the thoracic and lumbar spine are innervated by the same level and level above. The one notable exception is the L5–S1 joint, which receives innervation from the medial branch of L4 and the dorsal ramus of L5 [3].

The lower cervical spine vertebrae (C3–7) have additional articulations called the uncovertebral joints, or joints of Luschka. These joints are common locations of osteoarthritis, which

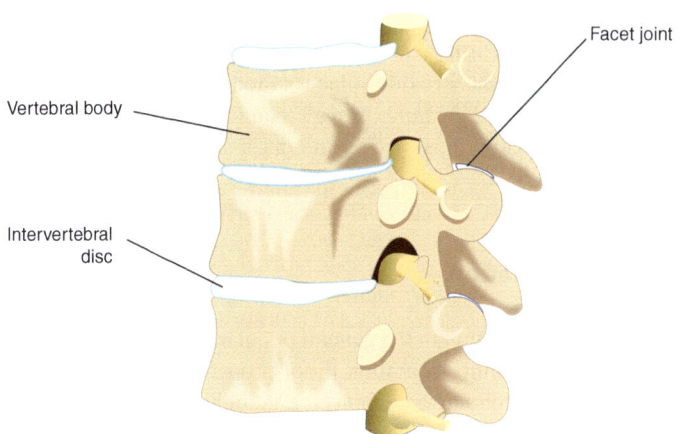

Fig. 3.1 Sagittal view of the spinal column depicting the vertebral body of the spinal cord, separated by intervertebral discs. Facet joints are formed between the articular processes of two adjacent vertebrae

narrows their corresponding intervertebral foramina. Thus, the most common locations of the cervical spine that exhibit degenerative changes are between C4–C7 [4].

Intervertebral or neural foramen are small openings between adjacent segments that serve as the exit site of the corresponding spinal nerve root. The foramen directly abut both the intervertebral disc and facet joint. Spinal ligaments run longitudinally, serving as strong fibrous bands that stabilize the spine. The three major ligaments are the anterior longitudinal ligament (ALL), posterior longitudinal ligament (PLL), and ligamentum flavum.

The intervertebral disc is composed of a viscous inner nucleus pulposus and outer annulus fibrosus. The nucleus pulposus is a gelatinous structure that is 90% water at birth. The annulus fibrosus consists of type I collagen fibers arranged obliquely that are anchored onto vertebral endplates. This fiber arrangement allows the annulus to withstand motion in most planes, but places it at risk for torsional injuries. A major function of the disc is shock absorption. The liquid nucleus pulposus is predominantly incompressible, and disc pressure subsequently results in stretching of the annulus fibers.

Discs Under Pressure
While facet joints provide some rotational resistance with a neutral spine, they cannot provide counterpressure with the spine in flexion, thus placing the discs at increased risk in this position.

3.1.2   Evaluation

While highly common in the general population, back pain can be a long-term disabling condition if not properly addressed. When evaluating this condition in gamers, a thoughtful and precise history and physical examination coupled with ergonomic assessment can provide sufficient clues to determine the etiology.

Mechanical Back Pain
Accounting for the majority of acute low back pain, mechanical pain refers to disruption in the inherent biodynamics of the anatomical components of the back.

3.1.2.1 History Taking
The esports history taking does not stray far from traditional pain evaluations. In addition to onset, timing, provocative, and palliative components and associated symptoms, special attention should be made for any red flags of a more malignant etiology. Patients with weakness may not simply state, "I have hand weakness", but express difficulty with buttons, mouse or controller grip, sluggishness with keyboard controls, or switching to new keybinds. The presence of numbness and tingling should always be further investigated to determine if symptoms fall in a specific peripheral nerve or dermatomal distribution.

Back Pain Red Flags
Pain associated with weakness, gait difficulties, or bladder and bowel dysfunction should be causes for concern, and suggest a myelopathic origin. Weight loss and systemic symptoms such as fever may point towards underlying malignancy.

3.1.2.2 Physical Examination

The esports examination should start with observation, both standing and seated. Examiners should pay special attention for any changes in spinal curvature or imbalances that may result from chronic maladaptive postures. Palpation may reveal hypertonic musculature, or active trigger points. Involved areas should be ranged both passively and actively to diagnose motion restrictions.

A thorough neurological examination should be incorporated into any evaluation of complaints with potential spinal origin including manual muscle testing, sensation, reflexes, and gait.

As with any other joint evaluation, the areas above and below should also be carefully investigated. For patients with neck pain, the shoulder should be evaluated for a referred pain origin. Similarly, the hip should be examined for patients with lower back complaints. If possible, visualization of the patient in their native gaming setup, either in real time or via photograph or teleconference, can reveal other imbalances.

3.1.2.3 Diagnostic Imaging

A large majority of neck and back complaints in the esports athlete may be diagnosed based on history and physical examination alone [6]. If further diagnostic workup is required, simple X-ray is often the first modality. However, advanced imaging may be an appropriate subsequent step if the patient:

1. Presents with clinical signs of cord compression or myelopathy
2. Does not respond to conservative treatment
3. Has findings other than age-appropriate changes on X-ray

Plain Radiography

X-rays are often the first and only imaging necessary in most cases of back and neck pain. Spine radiographs should consist of an anterior-posterior and lateral view. Lateral views may reveal signs of chronic poor posture, such as straightened, worsened, or reversed normal curvatures. Flexion/extension views are usually only necessary if instability is suspected, and oblique views can be obtained to examine for spondylolysis.

Magnetic Resonance Imaging

While almost never the most appropriate first test, MRI can be the most informative. MRI can reveal disc herniations, degenerative disc disease, and evidence of radiculopathy. Contrast is usually only required when tumor or infection is suspected.

While MRI may be beneficial in providing possible etiologies of symptoms, imaging may not correlate entirely with symptomatology. There is a very high incidence of positive findings on MRI in asymptomatic individuals. MRI results must be interpreted in conjunction with history and physical examination findings [6].

Computed Tomography (CT)

Despite being one of the best imaging modalities to evaluate facet joint pathology, CT is not often utilized. The use of CT imaging in the gaming population should be reserved for patients who cannot undergo MRI.

Electrodiagnostics

Nerve conduction studies (NCS) and electromyography (EMG) can be helpful in cases of peripheral neuropathy and radiculopathy. NCS can distinguish between peripheral neuropathies and more central etiologies. EMG can be very helpful in picking up early signs of denervation and subclinical weakness. Screening EMG to include six upper limb muscles and the appropriate cervical paraspinal level can successfully diagnose 94–99% of cervical radiculopathies [7]. The downside of EMG is largely patient discomfort. NCS involves repetitive electrical shocks, and EMG is performed via needle evaluation, and can be poorly tolerated. The patient should be educated on the testing procedure when it is prescribed, and not upon arrival to the testing facility.

3.1.3 Treatment

The exact treatment of a condition should obviously be reliant upon the underlying etiology. We will briefly discuss commonly employed treatment strategies across a majority of conditions, and expound on details in each specific pathology category.

3.1.3.1 Therapeutic Modalities

Cold and heat therapy is often the first line employed by patients themselves, prior to presenting to the health care practitioner. Providing brief patient education on the effects of temperature on the inflammatory cascade can have long-lasting benefits. Cold therapy can reduce pain via vasoconstriction, decreased inflammation, and metabolic demand. Topical heat may facilitate pain relief by increased blood flow and elasticity of connective tissues [8].

The choice of temperature treatment is not set in stone. Generally, acute inflammatory processes are better influenced by cold, whereas chronic processes respond more appropriately to heat [9].

Nontraditional modalities such as acupuncture, yoga, and osteopathic manual therapy, may also be helpful.

3.1.3.2 Rehabilitation

During periods of pain, the natural human tendency is to rest. However, for most cases, overt bed rest should be limited and attention should still be paid to stretching exercise and resumption of normal activities as soon as possible. Bed rest may lead to prolonged recovery times, and even worsening of symptoms.

Once the acute pain phase has been completed, strengthening exercises may speed recovery. Even with the most motivated of populations, self-directed programs may not be as regular or effective as a formal course of physical therapy. Formal therapy programs may diagnose imbalances, provide further stabilization, improve flexibility, and promote proper posture.

Transcutaneous electrical nerve stimulation (TENS) is a readily available device that delivers electrical impulses via surface electrodes. Studies have shown that TENS may be effective for chronic pain treatment when used in conjunction with more traditional modalities [10].

3.1.3.3 Pharmacological Management

Use of over-the-counter (OTC) anti-inflammatory and analgesic medications can be widespread and pervasive in the athletic population. Given their readily accessible nature, the side effects of OTCs may not be widely known. Non-steroidal anti-inflammatory drugs (NSAIDs) such as ibuprofen and naproxen block the inflammatory cascade via inhibiting the activity of cyclooxygenase enzymes (COX 1 and/or 2). Long-term NSAID usage can have deleterious effects, such as gastrointestinal distress/damage and kidney dysfunction. NSAIDs may also interact with other medication metabolism.

Prescription medications may be necessary for acute or chronic therapy. Anticonvulsants and antidepressants can be helpful for chronic pain and neuropathic symptoms.

Opioids, powerful analgesic medications that can lead to tolerance, dependence, addiction, and death, may have utilization in cancer-related pain and other conditions, but will not be discussed.

3.1.3.4 Interventions

While most cases of neck and back pain may be adequately treated with more conservative methods, more advanced methods may be necessary.

Interventional spinal procedures, such as nerve blocks and corticosteroid injections, are performed using fluoroscopic guidance by highly trained physicians. Steroid injections are not recommended for long-term use due to the deleterious effects on healthy cartilage, bones, and tendons.

3.2   Myofascial Conditions

Myofascial pain syndrome, Trigger points

3.2.1   Overview

The initial presentation of musculoskeletal pain can be daunting, as it is associated with a broad differential. While a large number of cases may be due to underlying spinal abnormalities, myofascial pain has been shown to be the source of pain complaints in up to 30% of patients. Myofascial pain is characterized by taut bands in the muscle, called trigger points, that reproduce pain symptoms with palpation. It is a common and treatable cause of neck and back pain that can easily be addressed by most health care professionals.

In the esports population, sedentary lifestyles and maladaptive postures may lead to an increased risk of myofascial conditions and at an earlier age than the non-gaming, age-matched population.

3.2.2   Pathogenesis

Myofascial pain syndrome is a seemingly simple, yet remarkably complex disorder whose etiology is still actively debated. Despite this, there is a general literature consensus on certain aspects. The primary pain generator is a trigger point, a hypercontracted, palpable area of muscle that may be present in one or more places. Palpation of the site often results in pain in an anatomically separate location, which is classified as referred pain.

While the precise pathophysiology of trigger points still remains unclear, it appears to be mediated by a central mechanism with an additional component of peripheral sensitization via the dorsal horn. Sustained sarcomere contracture leads to reduced blood flow and metabolic alterations, which in turn increases release of inflammatory mediators. Furthermore, in vivo studies have shown altered gluconeogenesis pathways in trigger points when compared to normal tissue as well as increased levels of lactate, suggesting the area itself is ischemic in nature [11, 12].

Development of trigger points may be preceded by seemingly trivial insults such as a minor muscle strain, long gaming session, adjustment of peripherals, sustained low-level contractions from chronic overuse, poor posture, or sleeping habits.

3.2.3 Presentation

The presentation of a patient with myofascial pain syndrome may be indistinguishable initially from that of discogenic or radiculo-pathic origins. Pain is often acute in onset, and may or may not radiate. Patients may describe specific movements or positions that cause aggravation. Quality may vary from deep and achy to lightening or electric-like symptoms. For trigger points near mid-line, presentation may closely mimic that of facet syndrome. Occasionally, patients may state they can reproduce their symp-toms with palpation, offering excellent diagnostic insight.

Certain researchers further classify trigger points as "active" or "latent," with the former producing spontaneous pain, the latter not. Both may elicit uncomfortable sensations with palpation [13]. Palpation may also elicit autonomic symptoms [14].

3.2.4 Diagnosis

The diagnosis of myofascial pain is purely clinical, as there is no clear diagnostic testing. The most commonly utilized criteria to define trigger points was developed by Tough [15].

1. Tender spot in a taut band of skeletal muscle
2. Patient pain recognition
3. Predicted pain referral pattern
4. Local twitch response

Physical examination findings of a normal motor and sensory exam coupled with a palpable nodule that reproduces symptoms suggests a component of myofascial pain. Provocative testing for radiculopathy and facet-mediated pain should be negative, such as neural tension tests.

3.2.5   Treatment

Once the diagnosis of myofascial pain syndrome is made, equal attention should be paid to both resolution of pain symptoms and prevention of further recurrence.

3.2.5.1 Therapeutic Modalities

Treatments like massage and stretching that are known to increase blood flow have been proposed to address the underlying microcirculation restriction. However, it is unclear if a regional increase in blood flow will affect the microcirculation of the trigger point.

Manual therapeutic modalities have been shown to reduce pain associated with active trigger points. Of the proposed modalities, trigger point manual therapy, counterstrain, and muscle energy techniques may be the most promising. Trigger point manual therapy is performed by applying sustained digital pressure to the area of interest. The counterstrain and muscle energy techniques were first developed by osteopathic physicians, and utilize inherent muscle reflexes such as the muscle spindle and Golgi tendon reflex.

3.2.5.2 Pharmacological Management

Analgesics, anti-inflammatories, and topical creams may provide symptomatic relief but do not adequately address the underlying pathophysiology.

3.2.5.3 Interventions

Dry needling and trigger point injections have become widely acceptable forms of treatment. Needle-based treatments have been shown effective to release myofascial trigger points by eliciting a localized twitch response. A twitch response is a transient increase in muscle activity, and is considered to be a spinal reflex, as spinal cord transection between the brain and trigger point does not elicit a response. Relaxation after the twitch is thought to relieve capillary constriction, thus normalizing microcirculation [13]. Evidence has shown increased localized blood flow to trigger points after intervention [16]. Both injection techniques can be performed in office without specialized equipment, and are generally well-tolerated. When choosing between the two, it is important to note that dry needling was found to be as effective as using an injectable, but the latter resulted in less post-treatment soreness [17] Dry needling has been shown to result in sustained relief from pain for at least 6 weeks following intervention. Caution must be taken when treating the rhomboids, upper trapezius, and levator scapulae given the close proximity of lung tissue and risk of pneumothorax.

Trigger point injections can be performed by appropriately trained health care providers, and are not limited to physician-only. Due to the efficacy and ease of treatment for this performance-declining condition, medical providers associated with esports teams are encouraged to pursue training.

Other modalities, such as chemodenervation, electrical stimulation, cold laser therapy, and ultrasound therapy have been employed to treat myofascial pain with varying efficacy [13, 18].

3.3   Thoracic Outlet Syndrome

3.3.1   Overview

Thoracic outlet syndrome is a condition in which either neural or vascular structures are compressed as they exit the thoracic outlet in the cervicothoracobrachial region. The majority of cases are neurological (95–99%); a small minority of cases involve compromise of either arterial or venous structures.

Compression primarily occurs at one of three anatomical sites: the interscalene triangle, the costoclavicular triangle, and the subcoracoid or sub-pectoralis minor space. The interscalene triangle consists of the space between the anterior scalene muscle anteriorly, the middle scalene muscle posteriorly, and the medial surface of the first rib inferiorly. The costoclavicular triangle is bound by the middle third of the clavicle anteriorly, the first rib posteromedially, and the upper border of the scapula posterolaterally. The subcoracoid space is bordered by the coracoid process superiorly, the pec minor anteriorly, and ribs 2–4 posteriorly.

Less commonly, clavicular hypomobility or the presence of a cervical rib can cause compression of neurovascular structures.

3.3.2 Pathogenesis

In the absence of structural alterations, such as a cervical rib, transversocostal or costocostal fibrous anomalies, abnormalities of the insertion of the scalene muscles, cervicodorsal scoliosis, or congenital uni- or bilateral elevated scapulae, thoracic outlet syndrome derives from acquired or functional discrepancies.

In gaming, traumatic sources such as clavicle fracture, rib fracture, or whiplash/hyperextension neck injury are unlikely. Esports patients with thoracic outlet syndrome are more likely to develop the condition from repetitive stress injuries or postural factors resulting in closure of the three spaces outlined above. This closure can result directly from poor posture or from compensatory alterations to the muscles that border these spaces, such as scalene hypertrophy; decreased trapezius, levator scapulae, or rhomboid resting tong; or shortening of the scalenes, trapezius, levator scapulae, or pectoral muscles.

3.3.3 Presentation

Symptoms depend on the portion of the plexus involved and the type of thoracic outlet syndrome: arterial, venous, or neurogenic. Generally, thoracic outlet syndrome does not follow dermatomal or myotomal distributions unless there is concomitant nerve root involvement.

Patients with upper plexus involvement (C5–7) present with pain in the side of the neck, ear, and face that may radiate to the rhomboids and pectorals. Patients with lower plexus involvement (C8–T1) present with pain in the shoulder that radiates down the ulnar side of the forearm and into the fourth and fifth digits.

With arterial thoracic outlet syndrome, patients demonstrate the "Ps and Cs": pallor, paresthesias, pain, claudication, and cold intolerance. With venous thoracic outlet syndrome, patients report a feeling of heaviness and demonstrate edema and paresthesias.

With neurogenic thoracic outlet syndrome, patients may demonstrate Raynaud's phenomenon, but more commonly present with paresthesias, numbness, weakness, decreased fine motor skills, and occipital headaches.

3.3.4 Diagnosis

Given the similarity of its clinical presentation to other conditions, any diagnosis of thoracic outlet syndrome must involve excluding other possible diagnoses.

Electromyography and nerve conduction studies will usually show decreased ulnar **sensorial** but normal ulnar **motor** potentials with normal median **sensorial** potentials. Similarly, venography and arteriography can assist with the identification of venous and arterial thoracic outlet syndrome.

At least two positive clinical tests are recommended for diagnosis via clinical testing only. Common thoracic outlet syndrome clinical tests are listed in Table 3.1 with their sensitivities, specificities, and likelihood ratios where available.

3.3.5 Treatment

Conservative management including physical therapy should initially focus on symptom relief, followed by progression to exercises to address the tissues causing compression and limitation of

Table 3.1 Reliability of thoracic outlet syndrome clinical tests [19]

Test	Sensitivity (%)	Specificity (%)	LR+	LR-
Roos	52–84	30–100	1.2–5.2	0.4–0.53
Adson	79	74–100	3.29	0.28
Wright	70–90	29–53	1.27–1.49	0.34–0.57
Upper limb tension test	90	38	1.5	0.3

motion. This may include joint mobilization, soft tissue mobilization, postural correction exercises, stretching of the muscles comprising the thoracic outlet, and strengthening of the muscles that stabilize the shoulder girdle and costoclavicular space.

Studies are mixed with regard to the efficacy of botulinum injections to the anterior and middle scalenes. Some studies have found improvement in pain and spasm, while others have been inconclusive [20, 21].

In most cases, surgical intervention is not indicated unless conservative management has been ineffective, with the notable exception of cases of vascular thoracic outlet syndrome with limb-threatening complications.

3.4   Postural Dysfunctions

3.4.1   Forward Head Posture

Nerd neck, iHunch

3.4.1.1 Overview

Forward head posture refers to a pattern of upper thoracic and lower cervical flexion coupled with upper cervical and occipital extension. In and of itself, this posture is not necessarily pathologic and may be attributed to naturally occurring variations in craniovertebal or odontoid process angle. However, forward head posturing may also develop as a consequence of combined muscular weakness, muscular tightness, and abnormal spinal mobility [22]. When this exists in conjunction with pain or weakness, or when the curvature becomes more prominent over time, it is more likely to be a pathological variant.

Both computer and console gamers are at an increased risk given their prolonged sedentary activities, and may have already begun to adopt this posture outside of gaming on presentation.

3.4.1.2 Pathogenesis
In cases of accentuated thoracic kyphosis or lumbar lordosis, forward head posture may develop in a compensatory manner. However, it generally results from prolonged poor positioning. This may occur in sitting, standing, or lying. Any position where atlantoaxial extension and distal cervical flexion occur in conjunction can contribute to the development of this condition, including:

1. Mobile gaming
2. Texting posture maintained for long durations
3. Sleeping with elevated head
4. Slouched/slumped positioning

With regard to gaming populations, this posture is particularly visible in common sitting positions for console players (e.g., Super Smash Bros. Melee).

Longstanding maintenance of this posture results in alterations in muscle lengths and relationships. Functionally, semispinalis cervicis is weakened and lengthened while semispinalis capitis (bilateral action: cervical and atlantoaxial extension, unilateral action: contralateral head and neck rotation) is shortened and hyperactive. The longus cervicis or longus colli acts to limit lordosis as produced by the weight of the head and posterior cervical muscle contraction; in forward head posture, this muscle is shortened and tight. The longus capitis (bilateral action: flexion of cervical spine and head, unilateral action: ipsilateral lateral flexion and rotation of neck and head), however, is *lengthened* due to its insertion directly onto the occipital bone, rather than onto more distal points as for the longus cervicis.

3.4.1.3 Presentation

Forward head posture rarely exists in isolation. Given the interconnected nature of the spine, this particular condition is often found in conjunction with thoracic kyphosis and lumbar lordosis, which will be addressed in the next two sections of this chapter.

Patients with forward head posture will demonstrate decreased overall cervical lordosis with compensatory extension at the atlanto-occipital joint. The head is subsequently shifted forward, hence the name.

Patients with forward head posture may report a variety of symptoms, including

• Increased pain and fatigue of neck and back muscles
• Decreased head and neck movement
• Tension headaches
• Jaw pain and inflammation
• Temperature changes in upper extremities
• Decreased arm and shoulder mobility
• Difficulty breathing
• Upper back/scapular pain

3.4.1.4 Diagnosis

Diagnosis is purely clinical, with minimal utility of diagnostic measures like ultrasonographic assessment of neck flexor and extensor muscles.

Any diagnosis of forward head posture should begin with observational postural analysis of the entire spine, given the interaction between the lumbar, thoracic, and cervical components. This assessment should be completed both in sitting, to assess patients in the positions assumed for gaming, and in standing, which is more sensitive to identification of forward head posture [23]. Traditionally employed by builders, a plumb line (a long string hanging from the ceiling with a weight attached to the end) can further aid diagnosis if available, as shown in Fig. 3.2.

Ergonomic assessment of an individual's setup should be conducted, as this is most often either the causative factor or aggravating factor.

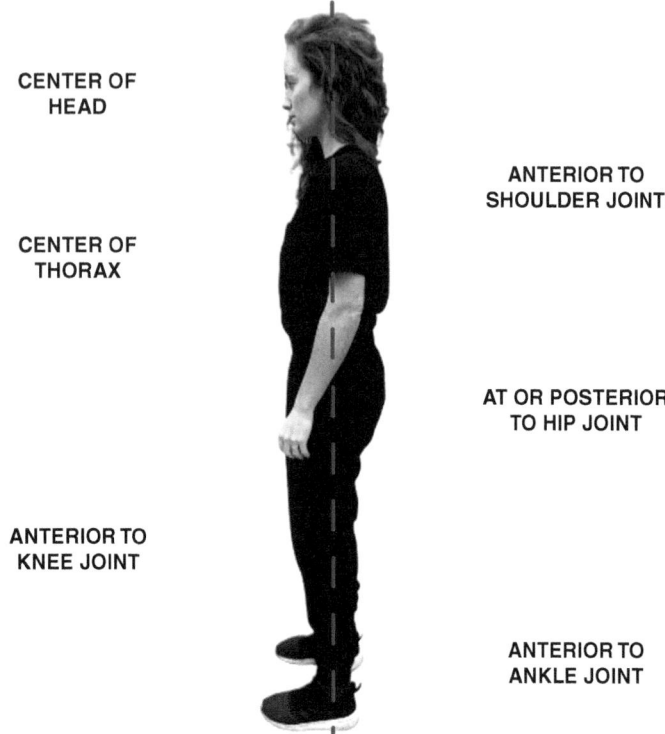

CENTER OF
HEAD

CENTER OF
THORAX

ANTERIOR TO
KNEE JOINT

ANTERIOR TO
SHOULDER JOINT

AT OR POSTERIOR
TO HIP JOINT

ANTERIOR TO
ANKLE JOINT

Fig. 3.2 An imaginary plumb line hanging directly down from the ceiling can be used to aid examination. When the body is in ideal posture, gravity should pass through specific joints and areas of the body, thus allowing for a more quantitative analysis

3.4.1.5 Treatment

Optimal treatment of forward head posture must be multifactorial to successfully address both the causative factors and underlying pathology. Any intervention to address musculoskeletal deficits will inevitably fail if not coupled with environmental alterations to support improved posture, including improved workspace and sleep ergonomics.

Table 3.2 Physical therapeutic interventions to target forward head posture

Posture	Cervical retraction
	Scapular retraction
Mobility/ flexibility	Cervical active/passive range of motion exercises
	Shoulder active/passive range of motion exercises
	Stretching of tight structures (most commonly trapezius, scalenes, sternocleidomastoid, pectoralis major/minor)
	Cervical self-SNAGs
Strength/ endurance	Cervical strengthening, progressing from isometric to isotonic
	Rhomboid/middle trapezius strengthening

Treatment of this condition is largely dependent on observed impairments, but will likely include the protocols listed in Table 3.2.

Manual therapy should be used to complement active exercises, but must be partnered with education for patients on the role of exercise for long-term improvement. Soft tissue mobilization to tight structures, including the cervical extensors, trapezius, scalenes, sternocleidomastoid, and pectoralis major and minor muscles, can supplement stretching exercises. In particular, myofascial release and occipital release can improve tightness and pain.

If intervertebral mobility is found to be lacking, central or unilateral posterior-anterior mobilization of the cervical spine may be appropriate. For patients with limited cervical rotation and facet joint mobility, sideglides, downglides, or SNAGs (sustained natural apophyseal glides) are appropriate. While research indicates that mobilization, thrust manipulation, and SNAGs all provide pain relief and improved mobility, they are not by themselves sufficient to resolve forward head posture [24]. Both cervical and thoracic mobilizations and thrust manipulations are correlated with short-term improvements in patients with mechanical neck pain. However, thoracic and cervical exercises supplemented with joint mobilizations are the most effective intervention for short- and long-term relief [25–27].

As with other myofascial conditions, electrical stimulation and thermal modalities may provide local, short-term pain relief but will not address underlying causes.

3.4.2 Excessive Thoracic Kyphosis

3.4.2.1 Overview
This overview is not designed to address structural issues of the thoracic spine, such as scoliosis, but rather excessive *postural* kyphosis deriving from a functional basis. This postural deficit is often associated with excessive cervical extension, or forward head posture, and can result from poor gaming ergonomics.

3.4.2.2 Pathogenesis
Postural kyphosis is most commonly a function of sustained poor positioning, leading to tight chest wall muscles, including pectoralis major and minor; weakened/lengthened thoracic extensors and scapular retractors; and decreased thoracic intervertebral mobility [28].

Excessive kyphosis may act as a compensatory mechanism for other postural deficits. Facet arthropathy, spondylitic changes, and disc degeneration may also promote excessive kyphosis as a pain-relieving mechanism.

3.4.2.3 Presentation
This condition is attributable to a pattern of weakness and tightness in the muscles of the chest and upper back. Patients will demonstrate a slumped or rounded upper back posture, often with scapular protraction and rounding of the shoulders as well. Patients often report feelings of fatigue, strain, or stiffness in the upper back.

The mobility of the thoracic spine subsequently affects the mobility of the shoulders, particularly at the scapulothoracic joint. Any report of limited shoulder mobility or pain in the shoulders should prompt clinicians to examine the thoracic spine as well.

3.4.2.4 Diagnosis
As with forward head posture, clinical examination is the primary means of identifying the underlying causes. Radiographic imaging may be useful to identify contributions from altered disc

height, osteophyte formation, facet joint changes, or vertebral fractures.

Of note, cervical spinal conditions commonly refer pain to the thoracic spine. As such, any examination for suspected thoracic pathology should also screen the cervical spine, particularly when the pain is located in the shoulder and scapular area.

3.4.2.5 Treatment

Ergonomic assessment and modification is key to prevention and continued support of good posture.

Limited research exists on the efficacy of spinal manipulation for thoracic musculoskeletal pain. Evidence does exist that spinal manipulation is associated with small, subclinical pain reductions and that multimodal care, including manual therapy, exercises, and education, is the most effective for pain reduction [29]. Research also suggests that changes in pain and mobility are greatest in patients who express positive perceptions of effect, further emphasizing the importance of education in clinical care.

Exercises should address patient-specific impairments and may include those described in Table 3.3.

Table 3.3 Physical therapeutic interventions to target excessive thoracic kyphosis

Posture	Scapular retraction Scapular retraction with external rotation Rows Seated thoracic extension
Mobility/ flexibility	Stretching of tight structures (most commonly pec major and minor) Thoracic self-mobilization with foam roller Prone press-ups Thoracic rotation/"open book" stretches Facilitated/segmental breathing
Strength/ endurance	Rhomboid/middle trapezius Core Latissimus dorsi Serratus anterior

3.4.3 Limited Lumbar Lordosis

While excessive lumbar lordosis can promote compensatory thoracic kyphosis, decreased lordotic curve is more closely associated with low back pain.

3.4.3.1 Overview

The mobility, stability, and positioning of the lumbar spine are all significantly impacted by the mobility, stability, and positioning of the hips, pelvis, and thoracic spine. In particular, limited hamstring flexibility has been found to correspond with limited lumbar lordosis and increased low back pain [30]. While limited data exist on posture within the gaming populations, analogous data from office workers who spend similar amounts of time sitting can provide a useful basis to draw conclusions about the role of posture in limiting lumbar lordosis and increasing risk for low back pain.

Environmental Factors
In addition to musculoskeletal factors, low back pain is highly correlated with depression, anxiety, work stress, and similar psychosocial factors. Current best practice for non-specific low back pain includes education and stress management techniques in addition to addressing relevant musculoskeletal factors [31].

3.4.3.2 Pathogenesis

As with forward head posture and excessive thoracic kyphosis, alterations in normal lumbar spine lordosis seen in gaming populations are most commonly attributable to chronic sub-optimal postures. The lumbar spine, as with the thoracic and cervical spine, is supported by a variety of passive (vertebrae, discs, joints, ligaments) and active (global and local muscles) structures that act together to provide stability and mobility. Coordination between active and passive structures is required to maintain normal curvature. Discoordination can result from a number of sources, including acute trauma, chronic disuse of active support structures (decreased engagement of core muscles), and chronic malpositioning of passive support structures (sustained poor posture).

3.4.3.3 Presentation

Patients with decreased lumbar lordosis may be largely asymptomatic. If pain is experienced, it is most often reported centralized over the lumbar spine, distributed across the pelvic brim, or in the muscles on either side of the lumbar spine. Patients may find relief in positions of increased hip and non-weight-bearing lumbar flexion.

3.4.3.4 Diagnosis

As with all postural conditions, observational postural analysis is the first step to identification of this condition. Clinicians should consider a variety of differential diagnoses and be aware that excessive lumbar lordosis is as likely to be a symptom as it is a cause of low back pain.

Radiographic imaging may be helpful to identify any structural changes. As with forward head posture and excessive thoracic kyphosis, decreased lumbar lordosis is often more of a functional than structural change. As such, clinical examination is the primary diagnostic tool for this particular postural impairment.

3.4.3.5 Treatment

Ergonomic assessment and modification is key to prevention of injury and continued support of good posture. Environmental modification and education should be part of any treatment plan for a patient with a postural dysfunction.

Depending on the primary cause, research suggests that conservative measures including physical therapy, cortisone injections, non-steroidal anti-inflammatory medications, and antidepressants are among the most effective treatments. Surgery is unlikely to be the best course of action barring serious structural concerns [31].

Treatment should emphasize continued mobility and avoidance of bedrest. A physical therapy plan to address low back pain

Table 3.4 Physical therapeutic interventions to target limited lumbar lordosis

Posture	Repeated/sustained lumbar extension exercises
	Anterior pelvic tilts
Mobility/flexibility	Hamstring stretching
	Hip internal/external rotation stretching
	Quadratus lumborum stretching
	ITB/TFL stretching
	Piriformis stretching
	Lumbar self-mobilization with foam roller
	Prone press-ups
Strength/endurance	Hip flexors
	Gluteus maximus and medius
	Quadriceps
	Lumbar extensors
	Core girdle

from decreased lumbar lordosis should address components discussed in Table 3.4.

3.5   The Spine

3.5.1   Spondylosis

Facet syndrome, Facet arthropathy, Spine osteoarthritis, Degenerative Disc Disease

3.5.1.1 Overview

Spondylosis is a general term used to describe degenerative changes of the spinal column. With aging, degenerative bony changes are as commonplace and unavoidable as white hair or wrinkles, and may be of little clinical significance. However, due to predisposing factors, the gaming population may be at an increased risk for early degeneration and clinical complications.

Spondylolysis
Spondylolysis is a vertebral defect of the pars interarticularis, most often observed at the L5 level. This is commonly seen in the pediatric population who engage in sports with hyperextension forces, like gymnastics.

3.5.1.2 Pathogenesis

Age-related wear and tear is a natural process of aging as cartilage wears away and intervertebral discs dessicate. This process may be accelerated by repetitive trauma, poor posture, abnormal spinal curvatures, or any process that places increased levels of stress on the spine. While the facet joints and discs may be anatomically separate, they have a corollary biomechanical relationship.

Degenerative Cascade

Repetitive microtrauma to the intervertebral disc results in circumferential outer annular tears. This subsequently interrupts blood flow to the disc, further undermining the structural integrity. Circumferential tears then coalesce into radial tears, which affect the underlying nucleus pulposus. A biologically incompetent disc places increased loads on the neighboring facet joints, accelerating degeneration and resulting in synovitis. Facet joint irritation leads to abnormal motion, as well as hypertonicity of the surrounding muscles. Thinning of the intervertebral disc from cumulative stress and annular tears reduces the shock-absorbing properties, placing more load on the facet joints. This cascade then continues, as dysfunctional motion leads to further microtrauma, synovial hypertrophy, and increased capsular laxity [32].

In response to joint instability and the subsequent pathological motion, the body responds by laying down additional bone in areas of increased stress, such as the vertebral endplates and facet joints. The result of this process is spondylosis and can affect the vertebral bodies, facet joints, and neural foramina. Degenerative disc disease often accompanies spondylosis, and it can be difficult to separate the two entities.

Additional articulations in the lower cervical spine, called the uncovertebral joints, or joints of Luschka, are predisposed to osteoarthritis. Degeneration at these locations can further narrow corresponding intervertebral foramina. Thus, the most common locations of the cervical spine that exhibit degenerative changes are between C4–C7. In the lumbar spine, L4–5 and L5–S1 are the most commonly affected facet joints.

Posture and Degeneration

The direct role of abnormal posture on degeneration is hotly debated. Any provider who has been involved in the low back pain treatment process knows it is not only complicated, but often multifactorial. Certain biomechanical correlates have been associated with low back pain with sitting, including intradiscal pressure, segmental loading, and segmental flexion. Intradiscal measurements have shown increased pressures during sitting when compared to standing, and a further increase in pressure with poor posture. Similarly, increases in segmental loading and flexion have been shown with sitting [33]. Furthermore, studies on neck pain have shown that forward head posture has been shown to lead to degenerative changes in the cervical spine. The mechanism is thought to be secondary to excessive stretching of the capsular ligaments, resulting in decreased threshold of nerve endings and altering proprioception.

Regardless, scientific research states posture has a role in back health, and should be thoroughly evaluated and treated like any other contributing factor. Console gamers may theoretically be at an increased risk, as simple observational inferences reveal increased lumbar flexion when compared to PC gamers.

3.5.1.3 Presentation

As spondylosis is a general condition, symptoms can manifest from a variety of etiologies. Pains may be primarily facetogenic, or arise when pressure is begun to be placed on the spinal cord (spinal stenosis) or nerve roots (radiculopathy).

When symptoms are facetogenic, patients may complain of neck or back stiffness. Symptoms are usually worse in the morning and during activity. Facet pain may manifest locally, or be referred. Patients may be able to pinpoint specific locations, often posterolateral to the spinous processes, and use terms such as "deep" and "achy." However, spondylotic pain may be difficult to localize. Patients may also complain of referred pain, depending on location. If the cervical spine is affected, symptoms may refer to the shoulder, proximal limb, or occiput. Facet-mediated pain typically does not radiate past the shoulder, and is aggravated by rotation or flexion. C1–2 and C2–C3 levels can refer rostrally to the occiput, so patients may commonly present with unilateral headaches.

Cervicogenic Headaches
Cervicogenic headaches can result from a multitude of underlying spinal pathologies, including spondylosis. They are typically unilateral, and radiate from the posterior occiput in a "ram's horn" pattern.

Patients with lumbar facet pain may present with referred hip pain or leg pain. Pain that radiates passed the knee or elbow suggests another etiology besides facet-mediated pain, such as radiculopathy [34]. Spondylosis resulting in radiculopathy often results in primarily radiating, appendicular pain [35]. These etiologies will be discussed at length in future sections.

Facet Syndrome Versus Radiculopathy
Unlike radiculopathy, radiating pain from facet syndrome does not follow a dermatomal pattern.

3.5.1.4 Diagnosis

Physical Examination
One of the most frequent findings on physical examination is decreased range of motion of the spine. This is most pronounced

in extension, where facet loading is at its highest. Lateral bending may also be affected, whereas neck rotation may be spared, as cervical rotation is a predominant function of the upper cervical spine. In addition to stiffness resulting from pathological spinal segments, surrounding paraspinal musculature tightens and becomes hypertonic. As the disease progresses, osteophytes may proliferate, further limiting segmental motion. Extension of the corresponding spinal region may be limited if facets are involved, and may result in pain.

Facet joints can be palpated and may be tender. In the cervical spine, they lie approximately 1 in. lateral to the spinous processes. It is important for the overlying muscles to be relaxed, as tightened overlying musculature may make palpation difficult. Patients may be placed in the prone position for best results. Similarly, overlying paraspinal muscles can be felt for hypertonicity, tenderness, and spasm.

The cervical compression test is a nonspecific test for cervical spondylosis. To perform, the examiner first laterally flexes the patient's head before providing an axial load. Ipsilateral neck pain indicates a positive result. In the lumbar spine, the lumbar facet loading test is performed by placing the lumbar spine in extension and ipsilateral rotation. This motion increases forces on the posterior facet joints, and may reproduce facetogenic symptoms.

Lhermitte's sign, a test classically employed for multiple sclerosis, is also a nonspecific test for cervical spondylosis. The test is considered positive if a feeling of electrical shock is felt down the spine with rapid passive neck flexion. A positive test suggests an underlying cervical spine process.

Imaging

Most patients with spondylosis do not require further investigation than a careful history and physical examination. There is no specific imaging study for facet-mediated pain. When imaging is performed, it should be used only in careful conjunction with gathered information, as spondylotic changes can be present in asymptomatic individuals. While X-ray or MRI may reveal degenerative changes, this is not diagnostic. Depending on the age of the patient, correlation between imaging and clinical symptoms is poor. For older patients, degenerative changes of the spine may be normal findings. However, in the younger, gaming population early arthritis should be considered abnormal. Disc degeneration can be seen in greater than half of adults in their 30s, and may not correlate with symptoms.

X-ray imaging can aid in diagnosis, and may reveal loss of disc height, osteophyte formation, facet joint changes, and subsequent foraminal narrowing. The radiographic presence of spondylosis in a young gamer should be considered abnormal.

3.5.1.5 Treatment

Conservative treatment is the mainstay of spondylosis treatment. While no amount of stretching or physical therapy can reverse degenerative changes, it can prevent progression and alleviate symptoms. Patients should first be educated on proper ergonomics and lifestyle modifications. For cervical spondylosis, special attention should be paid to desk and monitor heights. For primarily lumbar complaints, attention should be paid to what type of chair is being used, and the dimensions. Further guidelines can be provided in the ergonomics chapter (Chap. 5). For patients with acute pain, treatment should first be focused on pain control before progressing to stabilization and restoration of function of the affected spine.

Therapeutic Modalities

Heat and cold treatments are commonly employed by patients. Superficial cryotherapy induced vasoconstriction, thus decreasing the presence of inflammatory mediators, and subsequently pain. Cervical orthoses, such as soft collars, have a limited role and should be avoided long term.

Physical therapy can be effective for restoring range of motion, and may incorporate decompressive therapies such as traction. Therapy may focus on postural modification, proprioception, core strengthening, and flexibility. In general, extension-based protocols should be avoided to avoid further aggravation of the facet joint. For patients with lumbar complaints, hamstring flexibility is paramount as tightness can accentuate lumbar lordosis. Similarly, osteopathic manual medicine may be helpful [36].

Pharmacologic Management

Over-the-counter NSAIDs may provide analgesic and anti-inflammatory relief by helping quell the underlying inflammatory process and lessen spondylosis-related neck and back pain. If patients complain of muscle spasms, muscle relaxants may be clinically appropriate.

Interventions

Interventions targeting the facet joint can often provide lasting pain relief, and avoid the systemic consequences of oral medications.

Fluoroscopic-guided corticosteroid injections

Nociceptive input to the zygapophyseal joint is provided via the medial branches of corresponding spinal segments, and can be blocked via multiple interventions. Longer-lasting medial branch neurotomy is performed via radiofrequency ablation (RFA). For those who do not respond to RFA, decompressive surgery or fusion may be necessary.

3.5.2   Intervertebral Disc Disease

Discogenic pain, degenerative disc disease

3.5.2.1 Overview

Disc disease is a pathological process that results in anatomical changes in the intervertebral discs. This most commonly results from degeneration, trauma, or a combination of both. Intervertebral (IV) discs serve a vital role in back health, and loss of disc integrity can have a drastic effect on the surrounding structures including the facet joints, spinal nerves, and the spinal cord itself.

Disc disease can be further classified into degenerative disc disease, disc disruption, and disc herniation [37].

3.5.2.2 Pathogenesis

Disc disease is unlikely to arise from one specific cause, but rather a build-up of multiple microtraumas. Over time, small factors contribute to discal degeneration, which then predisposes that level to further injury, such as disruptions and herniations.

The IV disc has two components: the gelatinous inner nucleus pulposus and tough outer annulus. The primary function of the IV disc is to relieve pressure on the vertebral bodies. Subsequently, excessive loads can lead to disc damage via increased and nonoptimal pressure.

Intradiscal pressure is influenced by posture, though the effect on back pain is still debated. Lumbar disc pressures are lowest when supine, and highest when seated with forward flexion and some degree of weight bearing [38–40]. Furthermore, with the spine in neutral or extension, the facet joints offer some degree of movement guidance. However, when the spine is in flexion, facets offer very little resistance, placing further pressure on the IV discs.

Disc disease usually begins with small annular tears that coalesce over time. Disc degeneration may begin insidiously from small microtraumas, but as tears compound, the fluidity of the nucleus pulposus and the integrity of the annulus is compromised. As the internal architecture of the disc degrades, there may be a noticeable loss of disc height, which leads to instability and propensity for further injury. Forward flexion places anterior pressure on the disc and results in posterior nucleus pulposus displacement. Excessive anterior loads may result in prolapse of the inner nucleus pulposus through the annular fibers [41, 42]. Trauma, usually a result of improper lifting techniques, can also lead to prolapse of the inner nucleus pulposus. Herniated disc material can have further clinical consequences via compression of the spinal cord or spinal nerves.

Types of Disc Disease

Disc disruption refers to degeneration of the internal disc architecture with little or no noticeable external deformation. This can lead to disc herniation, which is extrusion of disc material outside of its anatomical region.

Disc herniations most commonly occur at C5–6, L4–5, and L5–S1. Disc herniations can be classified according to their location as either posterolateral, lateral, or central. Depending on the location of the herniation, radiculopathy may result for either direct mechanical pressure or the corresponding inflammatory response.

Posterolateral/paramedian disc herniations are the most common in the lumbar spine, as the lateral fibers of the posterior longitudinal ligament are the thinnest. As the spinal nerve of that corresponding level has already exited the spinal column, posterolateral disc herniations can result in compression of traversing, lower spinal nerves. Central disc herniations result from posterior pressure, possibly compressing the spinal cord itself, resulting in myelopathy or cauda equina past the conus medullaris.

3.5.2.3 Presentation

Disc disease often results in pain which may be acute or chronic. Acute pain is often accompanied by a history of lifting, twisting, bending, or coughing that may or may not correspond with a sensation of "popping." However, many cases of disc herniation are spontaneous and may not have a noticeable origin. Symptoms are often worsened by holding the neck in one position for long periods of time, such as driving or gaming. For esports athletes that may have organizational backing including personal trainers, disc herniations may be more common at the beginning of the season when they transition from little physical activity to formal training.

Discogenic pain alone is usually axial. If disc damage results in herniations that compress spinal nerves, axial pain is accompanied by radicular symptoms of the corresponding nerve level, which is discussed later in the chapter. Symptoms are aggravated by movements that place pressure on the disc, such as forward flexion or Valsalva.

3.5.2.4 Diagnosis

Physical Examination

When discogenic pain is suspected, a thorough neurological examination can often diagnose the exact level of injury, without requiring advanced imaging. The area of maximal pain should be inspected. Overlying musculature may be hypertonic or spasmodic. Palpation of the region around the spinous process may elicit pain. Range of motion may also be limited secondary to pain, most commonly in flexion. If symptoms are solely discogenic, patients should not have radicular symptoms.

Strength and sensory examination can reveal if there is any spinal nerve involvement, as well as reflex testing. Large central disc herniations can result in signs of myelopathy, indicating an urgent workup is necessary.

Imaging

Imaging may be included in the initial examination if there are signs of neurological compromise. Simple X-rays may reveal decreased disc height, foraminal narrowing, and facet arthrosis. MRI findings can be supportive of the diagnosis, but should only be used in careful conjunction with the history and physical examination. Disc degeneration can be found in up to a large majority of asymptomatic individual MRI images [43].

Certain MRI findings, such as annular fissures and Schmorl's nodes, have been found to be of unclear clinical significance. Annular fissures, or tears, have been found to have no correlation with back pain in multiple studies. Schmorl's nodes represent nucleus pulposus herniations and are related to degenerative changes, but have been found to not be an independent risk factor for back pain [44]. Modic changes (endplate degeneration) may also be seen on MRI and are related to degenerative disc disease, but their clinical significance remains unknown.

3.5.2.5 Treatment

Multiple studies have shown that disc protrusions and extrusions spontaneously resolve without surgical treatment [45]. However, pain may be acute and interfere with activities of daily living, and therefore impede recovery. The goal of nonsurgical treatment should be to reduce disc irritation and return the patient to their prior level of functioning. Complete, prolonged bed rest should never be recommended, and patients should be encouraged to continue pain-free activities [46].

Therapeutic Modalities

Exercise has been associated with positive outcomes in the treatment of low back pain and should be initiated once pain is tolerable. In addition to back and core strengthening, motor retraining may be necessary. Specific types of exercise is patient-specific, depending on the type and location of disc herniation, and should be individually tailored. Lumbar stabilization may address training of the small muscles of the spine, such as the multifidi.

Aquatic therapy has various benefits related to the properties of water itself. Pool-based therapy reduces gravitational stress on the body and increases buoyancy. Water can also decrease stress via the gate theory from the direct sensory input. Studies have also found manual therapy via spinal manipulation to be more effective than placebo [47].

Pharmacological Management

There is no clear consensus regarding the exact agents and duration of pharmacological management. NSAIDs use is common in the back pain population, and may have been consumed extensively prior to presentation to the health care practitioner. The role of muscle relaxants also remains controversial, and should be reserved for patients with pain that affects sleep. Topical treatments, such as diclofenac gel and lidoderm patches, may not penetrate deep enough to be truly effective, but have minimal side effects when compared to the oral formulations.

For patients with severe cervical radicular pain, a short course of oral glucocorticoid therapy may be warranted. However, the data is limited [48].

Interventions

Spinal procedures, such as epidural steroid injections, have become the bread and butter of interventional spine practices. By injecting anesthetic and corticosteroid into the anterior epidural space, the posterolateral intervertebral disc is bathed in medication, and may reduce pain. However, the efficacy of epidural steroid injection for discogenic pain has not been studied to satisfaction [49, 50].

Intradiscal electrothermography annuloplasty has not been shown to be an effective form of treatment. Intradiscal treatments, such as electrothermal therapy and percutaneous disc compression, are less invasive than surgical options, and may be effective in relieving cervical radicular pain caused by intervertebral disc protrusions.

Surgical options may be pursued for patients with persistent pain after conservative options have been fully explored, but the literature lacks a clear consensus [51].

3.5.3 Radiculopathy

3.5.3.1 Overview

Radiculopathy is a pathologic process affecting a spinal nerve root resulting in physiologic dysfunction. Symptoms resulting from spinal nerve root irritation or damage are referred to as radicular pain, and can produce a multitude of other symptoms in that specific nerve's dermatome and myotome.

3.5.3.2 Pathogenesis

Spinal nerve roots are the fundamental connection between the central and peripheral nervous system. Small rootlets leave the spinal cord, and converge into common trunks. They then traverse the spinal canal before exiting the intervertebral foramina. Because of anatomical differences in structure and vascularity, spinal nerve roots are inherently less resilient than peripheral nerves [52].

Nerve root damage may arise from a multitude of causes, the two major etiologies being direct mechanical pressure or chemical irritation. Direct pressure can result from spondylotic changes or disc herniation.

In the cervical spine, root injury is most commonly caused by intervertebral disc herniations, followed by spondylitis changes, including degenerative changes at the uncovertebral joint.

Disc herniations can lead to radiculopathy either via mechanical compression or via an inflammatory response. Disc herniation is a very common cause of radiculopathy, even if imaging findings reveal no direct mechanical compression. The nucleus pulposus is usually sequestered inside the annular fibers. When exposed to the body's environment, it becomes highly antigenic, and stimulates an autoimmune inflammatory cascade. This causes swelling and dysfunction of the neighboring spinal nerves. Similarly, direct mechanical compression compromises the vascularity, inducing local ischemia and subsequently setting off an inflammatory cascade.

3.5.3.3 Presentation

Radicular pain differs from that of facet and discogenic origins in that limb pain may be more prominent than axial pain. Axial pain may only be a secondary issue, or absent entirely. Patients often present with pain, numbness, tingling, or weakness in the distribution of the affected nerve root.

Differentials of Radiculopathy
Radiculopathy resulting from disc herniation is often acute in onset, with patients able to pinpoint the symptom onset. Spondylotis-related radiculopathy is often more insidious in the onset.

Symptoms resulting from radicular pain depend on the level of the spinal nerve root involved. For lumbosacral involvement, over 90% are L5 and S1 radiculopathies. Patients may also present with sensory loss, weakness, and reflex changes in the specific nerve distribution. Patients may also present with the diagnosis of sciatica, a nonspecific term used to describe a variety of conditions in which the primary complaint is burning pain running in the general sciatic nerve distribution.

Sciatica
Most sciatica diagnoses can be credited to L5 or S1 radiculopathy rather than piriformis syndrome or other direct injuries to the sciatic nerve.

3.5.3.4 Diagnosis

Physical Examination
A diagnosis of radiculopathy is suspected if history taking reveals radiating appendicular pain that crosses more than two joints. A careful neurological evaluation may reveal subclinical abnormalities. Sensory evaluation may show specific dermatomal delineations, shown in Fig. 3.3. Localized muscle weakness may be elicited via manual muscle testing. Long-standing radiculopathy may result in muscle wasting of the corresponding myotome that is visible to the naked eye. Severe muscle weakness is unlikely related to a single nerve root pathology, and points towards another, more distal etiology. When lumbar radiculopathy is suspected, gait evaluation, including heel and toe walking, may show side-to-side differences. Single leg calf raises can also determine side-to-side differences in calf strength. Key reflexes, muscles, and their corresponding dermatomes are listed in Tables 3.5 and 3.6.

Root Tension Signs
After a neurological evaluation has been performed, specific provocative tests that place the nerve under traction offer further evidence [53]. By placing the spinal nerves under traction, symptoms attributed to radiculopathy may be reproduced.

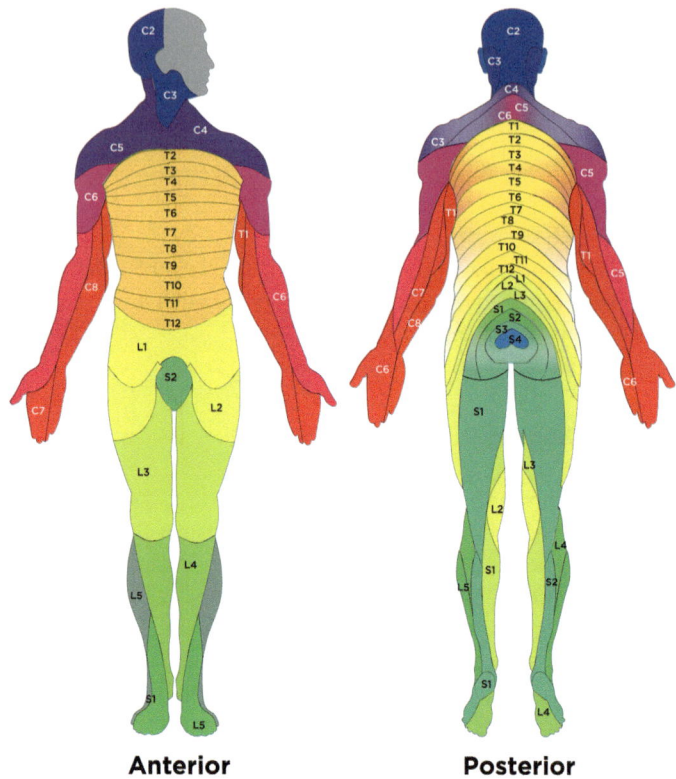

Fig. 3.3 Spinal dermatome map

Upper Limb Tension Test

The upper limb tension test (Elvey's Test) can aid in diagnosis of cervical radiculopathy. To perform the test, in a seated position, the patient's head is rotated contralaterally while the ipsilateral arm is abducted with the elbow in full extension. Symptom reproduction is considered a positive test.

Straight Leg Raise Test

Lumbar radiculopathy can be investigated using the straight leg raise (SLR) or slump test. The straight leg raise test, also known

Table 3.5 Cervical nerve roots and their corresponding dermatomes, key muscles, and associated reflexes

Root level	Dermatome	Key muscles	Reflexes
C5	Shoulder, lateral arm	Deltoid	Supinator
C6	Lateral forearm, thumb, and index finger	Biceps	Biceps
C7	Middle finger	Triceps	Triceps
C8	4th and 5th digits	Finger abduction	None
T1	Medial forearm	Intrinsic hand muscles	None

Table 3.6 Lumbar nerve roots and their corresponding dermatomes, key muscles, and associated reflexes

Root level	Dermatome	Key muscles	Reflexes
L1	Greater trochanter, groin	None	None
L2	Front of thigh	Psoas	None
L3	Front of thigh, medial lower leg	Quadriceps	Knee jerk
L4	Inner buttock, dorsum of foot, big toe	Tibialis anterior	Weak knee jerk
L5	Back of thigh, lateral leg, dorsum of foot	EHL	Hamstring
S1	Buttock, back of thigh	Calf	Ankle jerk

as Lasegue's test, has various protocols. In general, the test is performed with the patient in the supine position. The examiner flexes the patient's hip by lifting the affected leg from the table with the foot held in dorsiflexion. Reproduction of radiating symptoms is considered a positive test, and usually occurs when hip flexion is between 30° and 60°. A second, verification step, may be taken by flexing the knee. A bowstring sign refers to pain relief with a flexed knee during a positive straight leg raise test. The SLR test places the lumbosacral nerve roots under dural tension, and is most helpful for L5 and S1 radiculopathies [54].

Hamstring Tightness
Hamstring tightness is highly prevalent in the gaming population, and can lead to falsely positive SLR testing. Pain and tightness in the distribution of the hamstrings is not considered a positive test.

Slump Test
The slump test can offer further confirmation, and be helpful for patients who may not be able to assume the supine position. The seated patient is asked to slump forward with poor posture while the examiner extends the knee. Radiating pain down the sciatic nerve distribution is considered positive.

Reverse Straight Leg Test
Also known as the femoral nerve stretch test or Ely's test, this test is performed with the patient in the prone position and the examiner on the patient's affected side. The examiner then extends the hip with the knee held in 90 degrees of flexion. The test is considered positive if anterior thigh pain is felt, or symptoms are reproduced, and is suggestive of femoral nerve or L2–4 root involvement.

Spurling's Test
The traditional Spurling maneuver is formed by keeping the head in neutral and applying axial pressure from the top of the head down the cervical spine. However, the modified Spurling's maneuver (usually also referred to as "Spurling's maneuver") is more commonly employed. The patient is placed in cervical extension, and ipsilateral rotation and lateral bending. Axial pressure is then added. The test is considered positive if symptoms are reproduced and travel past the shoulder. Localized neck pain on testing is not considered positive. While the sensitivity of modified Spurling's is high, the sensitivity is unreliable. Thus, a negative test does not rule out cervical radiculopathy.

Distraction Tests
Shoulder Abduction Relief Sign
In a sitting position, the patient's ipsilateral humerus is abducted. Alleviation of radicular pain is considered positive.

Manual Neck Distraction Test
The manual neck distraction test is performed by applying superior traction at the base of the occiput and jaw. The test is considered positive if symptoms decrease.

Imaging
For the majority of atraumatic neck and back pain, imaging is not necessary. A 2009 meta-analysis compared immediate imaging with usual care for patients with acute to subacute back pain, and found no difference in long-term outcomes between the two groups [55].

X-Ray
If conservative treatment is ineffective, or patients describe pain affecting their ability to perform their activities of daily living or occupation, imaging may be pursued. In most cases, X-ray of the spine should be the first imaging study performed to evaluate radicular pain. Images may reveal degenerative changes of the spine, or facet narrowing. Spine radiographs should consist of an anterior-posterior and lateral view. Lateral views may reveal signs of chronic poor posture, such as straightened, worsened, or reversed normal curvatures. Flexion/extension views are usually only necessary if instability is suspected.

Magnetic Resonance Imaging
MRI is usually only necessary if the patient is not responsive to conservative treatment, if there is progression of symptoms, or X-ray reveals findings other than age-appropriate changes. MRI may be considered prior to X-ray if there are physical exam findings suggestive of cord compression or myelopathy. If MRI is contraindicated, CT myelography may be a suitable alternative.

Electrodiagnostics

Electrodiagnostic tests such as nerve conduction studies and electromyography can be used to distinguish cervical radicular pain from peripheral nerve entrapment or neuropathy. Screening EMG that includes six upper limb muscles and corresponding cervical paraspinal levels can identify 94–99% of cervical radiculopathies [7].

3.5.3.5 Treatment

Radiculopathy can often be extremely painful, and treatment should focus on symptomatic relief and resumption of ADLs. After acute pain has resolved, attention should be paid to find the underlying cause. Radiculopathy in the young population that is not related to improper lifting mechanics should always be considered abnormal. Due to poor posturing, the gaming population may be at an increased risk for spondylosis, disc degeneration, and subsequent radiculopathy. Prevention of future occurrences should be the final treatment step.

Therapeutic Modalities

Thermotherapy and cold therapy may be used to modulate pain. Deep heating modalities (ultrasound) are best avoided in the case of radiculopathy as this may increase inflammation and further aggravate the nerve root. TENS can assist in pain modulation, thus allowing patients to participate in more aggressive forms of therapy. TENS has been shown to be useful in certain instances of low back pain, and is believed to act via the gate theory. By stimulating large fibers, this blocks nociceptive input.

Cervical traction, application of a distracting force to the neck is commonly used for cervical radiculopathy, but lacks proven efficacy [56].

Patient education should be focused on assisting the patient in finding optimal pain-free positioning. Physical activity should be resumed as early as possible.

Physical therapy can be beneficial for not only pain resolution but prevention of further recurrences. Spinal biomechanics can be restored via diagnosis and treatment of range-of-motion deficits, and emphasis on strengthening and stabilization of related muscles.

Pharmacological Management

Oral NSAIDs are considered first-line pharmacological management for cervical radiculopathy. The clinical indications for lumbosacral involvement is less clear, as there is little evidence to suggest that NSAIDs are more effective to placebo in patients with sciatic distribution pain [57]. Adjunct medications may include muscle relaxants, tricyclic antidepressants, and antiepileptics. Muscle relaxants are best used in the acute period and at night due to their sedating side effects. Gabapentin is also commonly employed for the treatment of radicular pain. Gabapentin is best started at night due to sedating side effects, and gradually titrated up as tolerated. Pregabalin may also be used for those who do not tolerate gabapentin or hepatic or renal impairments [55]. Tricyclic antidepressants and SSRIs may also provide more long-term control of pain [58].

Interventions

Epidural steroid injections decrease inflammation through corticosteroid injection of nerve roots. The nerve root is bathed in corticosteroid solution in the epidural space. These treatments are effective for symptom management, and should be used only in combination with active rehabilitation [59].

The Spine Patient Outcome Research Trial found that surgery was favorable over nonoperative treatment in patients with lumbar radicular symptoms caused by disc herniation [60]. While surgery may lead to faster resolution of symptoms, long-term functional outcomes are similar to nonsurgical treatment options. Surgical intervention has not shown to have greater outcomes when compared with conservative measures. Surgical evaluation is considered prior to conservative management when there is evidence of progressive neurologic deficits [61].

References

1. Poquet N, Lin CWC, Heymans MW, van Tulder MW, Esmail R, Koes BW, et al. Back schools for acute and subacute non-specific low-back pain. Cochrane Database Syst Rev. 2016;4:CD008325. https://doi.org/10.1002/14651858.CD008325.pub2.
2. DiFrancisco-Donoghue J, Balentine J, Schmidt G, Zwibel H. Managing the health of the esport athlete: an integrated health management model. BMJ Open Sport Exerc Med. 2019;5:e000467. https://doi.org/10.1136/bmjsem-2018-000467.
3. Binder DS, Nampiaparampil DE. The provocative lumbar facet joint. Curr Rev Musculoskelet Med. 2009;2(1):15–24. https://doi.org/10.1007/s12178-008-9039-y.
4. Gilchrist RV, Slipman CW, Bhagia SM. Anatomy of the intervertebral foramen. Pain Physician. 2002;5(4):372–8.
5. Chou R, Fu R, Carrino JA, Deyo RA. Imaging strategies for low-back pain: systematic review and meta-analysis. Lancet 2009;373(9662):463–72. https://doi.org/10.1016/S0140-6736(09)60172-0.
6. Brinjikji W, Luetmer PH, Comstock B, Bresnahan BW, Chen LE, Deyo RA, et al. Systematic literature review of imaging features of spinal degeneration in asymptomatic populations. Am J Neuroradiol. 2015;36(4):811–6. https://doi.org/10.3174/ajnr.A4173.
7. Dillingham TR, Lauder TD, Andary M, Kumar S, Pezzin LE, Stephens RT, et al. Identification of cervical radiculopathies: optimizing the electromyographic screen. Am J Phys Med Rehabil. 2001;80(2):84–91. https://doi.org/10.1097/00002060-200102000-00002.
8. Malanga GA, Yan N, Stark J. Mechanisms and efficacy of heat and cold therapies for musculoskeletal injury. Postgrad Med. 2015;127(1):57–65. https://doi.org/10.1080/00325481.2015.992719.
9. Schmidt KL, Ott VR, Röcher G, Schaller H. Heat, cold and inflammation. Z Rheumatol. 1979;38(11–12):391–404.
10. Johnson M. Transcutaneous electrical nerve stimulation: mechanisms, clinical application and evidence. Rev Pain. 2007;1(1):7–11. https://doi.org/10.1177/204946370700100103.
11. Jafri MS. Mechanisms of myofascial pain. Int Sch Res Notices. 2014;523924. https://doi.org/10.1155/2014/523924.
12. Bron C, Dommerholt JD. Etiology of myofascial trigger points. Curr Pain Headache Rep. 2012;16(5):439–44. https://doi.org/10.1007/s11916-012-0289-4.
13. Gerber LH, Sikdar S, Aredo JV, Armstrong K, Rosenberger WF, Shao H, et al. Beneficial effects of dry needling for treatment of chronic myofascial pain persist for 6 weeks after treatment completion. PM R. 2017;9(2):105–12. https://doi.org/10.1016/j.pmrj.2016.06.006.

14. Shah JP, Thaker N, Heimur J, Aredo JV, Sikdar S, Gerber L. Myofascial trigger points then and now: a historical and scientific perspective. PM R. 2015;7(7):746–61. https://doi.org/10.1016/j.pmrj.2015.01.024.

15. Tough EA, White AR, Richards S, Campbell J. Variability of criteria used to diagnose myofascial trigger point pain syndrome – evidence from a review of the literature. Clin J Pain. 2007;23(3):278–86. https://doi.org/10.1097/AJP.0b013e31802fda7c.

16. Dommerholt J, Chou LW, Hooks T, Thorp JN. Myofascial pain and treatment: editorial a critical overview of the current myofascial pain literature. J Bodyw Mov Ther. 2019;23(4):773–84. https://doi.org/10.1016/j.jbmt.2019.10.001. Epub 2019 Oct 4

17. Alvarez DJ, Rockwell PG. Trigger points: diagnosis and management. Am Fam Physician. 2002;65(4):653–60.

18. Soares A, Andriolo RB, Atallah ÁN, da Silva EMK. Botulinum toxin for myofascial pain syndromes in adults. Cochrane Database Syst Rev. 2014;7:CD007533. https://doi.org/10.1002/14651858.CD007533.pub3.

19. Gillard J, Pérez-Cousin M, Hachulla É, Remy J, Hurtevent JF, Vinckier L, Thévenon A, Duquesnoy B. Diagnosing thoracic outlet syndrome: contribution of provocative tests, ultrasonography, electrophysiology, and helical computed tomography in 48 patients. Joint Bone Spine. 2001;68(5):416–24.

20. Finlayson HC, O'Connor RJ, Brasher PMA, Travlos A. Botulinum toxin injection for management of thoracic outlet syndrome: a double-blind, randomized, controlled trial. 2011;152(9):2023–8. https://doi.org/10.1016/j.pain.2011.04.027.

21. Christo PC, Christo DK, Carinci AJ, Freischlag JA. Single CT-guided chemodenervation of the anterior scalene muscle with botulinum toxin for neurogenic thoracic outlet syndrome. Pain Med. 2010;11(4):504–11. https://doi.org/10.1111/j.1526-4637.2010.00814.x.

22. Koseki T, Kakizaki F, Hayashi S, Nishida N, Itoh M. Effect of forward head posture on thoracic shape and respiratory function. J Phys Ther Sci. 2019;31(1):63–8. https://doi.org/10.1589/jpts.31.63.

23. Shaghayegh Fard B, Ahmadi A, Maroufi N, Sarrafzadeh J. Evaluation of forward head posture in sitting and standing positions. Eur Spine J. 2015;25(11):3577–82. https://doi.org/10.1007/s00586-015-4254-x.

24. Lopez-Lopez A, Alonso Perez JL, González Gutierez JL, La Touche R, Lerma Lara S, Izquierdo H, et al. Mobilization versus manipulations versus sustain apophyseal natural glide techniques and interaction with psychological factors for patients with chronic neck pain: randomized controlled trial. Eur J Phys Rehabil Med. 2015;51(2):121–32.

25. Im B, Kim Y, Chung Y, Hwang S. Effects of scapular stabilization exercise on neck posture and muscle activation in individuals with neck pain and forward head posture. J Phys Ther Sci. 2015;28(3):951–5.

26. Sheikhhoseini R, Shahrbanian S, Sayyadi P, O'Sullivan K. Effectiveness of therapeutic exercise on forward head posture: a systematic review and

meta-analysis. J Manip Physiol Ther. 2018;41(6):530–9. https://doi.
org/10.1016/j.jmpt.2018.02.002.

27. Cho J, Lee E, Lee S. Upper thoracic spine mobilization and mobility
exercise versus upper cervical spine mobilization and stabilization exercise in individuals with forward head posture: a randomized clinical trial.
BMC Musculoskelet Disord. 2017;18(1):525. https://doi.org/10.1186/
s12891-017-1889-2.

28. Sahrmann S. Movement system impairment syndromes of the extremities, cervical and thoracic spines. New York: Elsevier Health Sciences;
2010.

29. Southerst D, Marchand AA, Côté P, Shearer HM, Wong JJ, Varatharajan
S, et al. The effectiveness of noninvasive interventions for musculoskel-
etal thoracic spine and chest wall pain: a systematic review by the Ontario
Protocol for Traffic Injury Management (OPTIMa) collaboration. J
Manip Physiol Ther. 2015;38(7):521–31. https://doi.org/10.1016/j.
jmpt.2015.06.001.

30. Sadler SG, Spink MJ, Ho A, De Jonge XJ, Chuter VH. Restriction in lateral bending range of motion, lumbar lordosis, and hamstring flexibility
predicts the development of low back pain: a systematic review of prospective cohort studies. BMC Musculoskelet Disord. 2017;18(1):179.
https://doi.org/10.1186/s12891-017-1534-0

31. Delitto A, George S, Van Dillen L, Whitman JM, Sowa G, Shekelle P,
et al. Low back pain: clinical practice guidelines linked to the international classification of functioning, disability, and health from the ortho-
paedic section of the American Physical Therapy Association. J Orthop
Sports Phys Ther. 2012;42(4):A1–A57. https://doi.org/10.2519/
jospt.2012.42.4.A1

32. Kalichman L, Hunter DJ. Lumbar facet joint osteoarthritis: a review.
Semin Arthritis Rheum. 2007;37(2):69–80. https://doi.org/10.1016/j.
semarthrit.2007.01.007.

33. Hedman TP, Fernie GR. Mechanical response of the lumbar spine to
seated postural loads. Spine. 1997;22(7):734–43. https://doi.
org/10.1097/00007632-199704010-00004.

34. Schwarzer AC, Wang SC, Bogduk N, McNaught PJ, Laurent
R. Prevalence and clinical features of lumbar zygapophysial joint pain:
a study in an Australian population with chronic low back pain. Ann
Rheum Dis. 1995;54:100–6. https://doi.org/10.1136/ard.54.2.100.

35. Binder A. Cervical spondylosis and neck pain. Br Med J.
2007;334(7593):527–31. https://doi.org/10.1136/bmj.39127.608299.80.

36. Bronfort G, Haas M, Evans RL, Bouter LM. Efficacy of spinal manipulation and mobilization for low back pain and neck pain: a systematic
review and best evidence synthesis. Spine J. 2004;4:335–56. https://doi.
org/10.1016/j.spinee.2003.06.002.

37. Fardon DF, Williams AL, Dohring EJ, Murtagh FR, Gabriel Rothman
SL, Sze GK. Lumbar disc nomenclature: version 2.0: recommendations

of the combined task forces of the North American Spine Society, the American Society of Spine Radiology, and the American Society of Neuroradiology. Spine. 2014;39(24):E1448–65. https://doi.org/10.1097/BRS.0b013e3182a8866d.

38. Wilke HJ, Neef P, Caimi M, Hoogland T, Claes LE. New in vivo measurements of pressures in the intervertebral disc in daily life. Spine. 1999;24(8):755–62. https://doi.org/10.1097/00007632-199904150-00005.

39. Claus A, Hides J, Moseley GL, Hodges P. Sitting versus standing: does the intradiscal pressure cause disc degeneration or low back pain? J Electromyogr Kinesiol. 2008;18(4):550–8. https://doi.org/10.1016/j.jelekin.2006.10.011.

40. Bogduk N, Windsor M, Inglis A. The innervation of the cervical intervertebral discs. Spine. 1988;13(1):2–8. https://doi.org/10.1097/00007632-198801000-00002.

41. Choi YS. Pathophysiology of degenerative disc disease. Asian Spine J. 2009;3(1):39–44. https://doi.org/10.4184/asj.2009.3.1.39.

42. Munter FM, Wasserman BA, Wu HM, Yousem DM. Serial MR imaging of annular tears in lumbar intervertebral disks. AJNR Am J Neuroradiol. 2002;23(7):1105–9.

43. Jarvik JJ, Hollingworth W, Heagerty P, Haynor DR, Deyo RA. The Longitudinal Assessment of Imaging and Disability of the Back (LAIDBack) Study: baseline data. Spine. 2001;26(10):1158–66. https://doi.org/10.1097/00007632-200105150-00014.

44. Yin R, Lord EL, Cohen JR, Buser Z, Lao L, Zhong G, et al. Distribution of Schmorl nodes in the lumbar spine and their relationship with lumbar disk degeneration and range of motion. Spine. 2015;40(1):E49–53. https://doi.org/10.1097/BRS.0000000000000658.

45. Saal JS, Saal JA, Yurth EF. Nonoperative management of herniated cervical intervertebral disc with radiculopathy. Spine. 1996;21(16):1877–83. https://doi.org/10.1097/00007632-199608150-00008.

46. Hagen KB, Hilde G, Jamtvedt G, Winnem M. Bed rest for acute low-back pain and sciatica. Cochrane Database Syst Rev. 2004;4:CD001254. https://doi.org/10.1002/14651858.CD001254.pub2.

47. Assendelft WJ, Morton SC, Yu EI, Suttorp MJ, Shekelle PG. Spinal manipulative therapy for low back pain. Cochrane Database Syst Rev. 2004;1:CD000447. https://doi.org/10.1002/14651858.CD000447.pub2.

48. Ghasemi M, Masaeli A, Rezvani M, Shaygannejad V, Golabchi K, Norouzi R. Oral prednisolone in the treatment of cervical radiculopathy: a randomized placebo controlled trial. J Res Med Sci. 2013;18(Suppl 1):S43–6.

49. Vallée JN, Feydy A, Carlier RY, Mutschler C, Mompoint D, Vallée CA. Chronic cervical radiculopathy: lateral-approach periradicular corticosteroid injection. Radiology. 2001;218(3):886–92. https://doi.org/10.1148/radiology.218.3.r01mr17886.

50. Bush K, Hillier S. Outcome of cervical radiculopathy treated with periradicular/epidural corticosteroid injections: a prospective study with independent clinical review. Eur Spine J. 1996;5(5):319–25. https://doi.org/10.1007/bf00304347.

51. Manchikanti L, Helm S, Singh V, Benyamin RM, Datta S, Hayek SM, Fellows B, Boswell MV. An algorithmic approach for clinical management of chronic spinal pain. Pain Physician. 2009;12(4):E225–64.

52. Olmarker K. Spinal nerve root compression. Acta Orthop Scand. 1991;62(Suppl 242):1–27. https://doi.org/10.3109/17453679109153920.

53. Thoomes EJ, van Geest S, van der Windt DA, Falla D, Verhagen AP, Koes BW, et al. Value of physical tests in diagnosing cervical radiculopathy: a systematic review. Spine J. 2018;18(1):179–89. https://doi.org/10.1016/j.spinee.2017.08.241.

54. Kamath SU, Kamath SS. Lasègue's sign. J Clin Diagn Res. 2017;11(5):RG01–2. https://doi.org/10.7860/JCDR/2017/24899.9794.

55. Chou R, Huffman LH. Medications for acute and chronic low back pain: a review of the evidence for an American Pain Society/American College of Physicians clinical practice guideline. Ann Intern Med. 2007;147(7):505–14. https://doi.org/10.7326/0003-4819-147-7-200710020-00008.

56. Graham N, Gross AR, Goldsmith C. Mechanical traction for mechanical neck disorders: a systematic review. J Rehabil Med. 2006;38(3):145–52. https://doi.org/10.1080/16501970600583029.

57. Rasmussen-Barr E, Held U, Grooten WJ, Roelofs P, Koes B, van Tulder M, Wertli M. Non-steroidal anti-inflammatory drugs for sciatica. Cochrane Database Syst Rev. 2016;10(10):CD012382. https://doi.org/10.1002/14651858.CD012382.

58. Chiodo A, Haig AJ. Lumbosacral radiculopathies: conservative approaches to management. Phys Med Rehabil Clin N Am. 2002;13(3):609–21, viii. https://doi.org/10.1016/s1047-9651(02)00021-9.

59. Anderberg L, Annertz M, Persson L, Brandt L, Säveland H. Transforaminal steroid injections for the treatment of cervical radiculopathy: a prospective and randomised study. Eur Spine J. 2007;16(3):321–8. https://doi.org/10.1007/s00586-006-0142-8.

60. Weinstein JN, Lurie JD, Tosteson TD, Tosteson AN, Blood EA, Abdu WA, et al. Surgical versus nonoperative treatment for lumbar disc herniation: four-year results for the Spine Patient Outcomes Research Trial (SPORT). Spine. 2008;33(25):2789–800. https://doi.org/10.1097/BRS.0b013e31818ed8f4.

61. Schoenfeld AJ, Weiner BK. Treatment of lumbar disc herniation: evidence-based practice. Int J Gen Med. 2010;3:209–14. https://doi.org/10.2147/ijgm.s12270.

Lower Extremity Disorders in Esports

4

Caitlin McGee

4.1 General

While gamers rely on their lower extremities to a considerably lesser degree than their traditional sport counterparts, they still remain susceptible to certain disorders. Unlike the upper extremity, lower extremity injuries in esports are less commonly the result of repetitive microtrauma and more commonly the result of prolonged and sustained seated positioning.

Given that gamers are significantly more conscious of the importance of their hands, one of the primary barriers to treatment of lower extremity injuries and disorders in the competitive gaming population is a lack of understanding. Education is a crucial component of any rehabilitation program, but particularly so here. A thorough understanding of the provoking factors – How long does the player sit for? On what surface? What activities do they engage in outside of gaming? How often? – is also essential for appropriate intervention, which is likely to include ergonomic modification as appropriate (Chap. 5).

C. McGee (✉)
1HP, Washington, DC, USA

© The Author(s), under exclusive license to Springer Nature Switzerland AG 2021
L. Migliore et al. (eds.), *Handbook of Esports Medicine*,
https://doi.org/10.1007/978-3-030-73610-1_4

119

4.1.1   Anatomy

The lower extremity includes structures from the hip to the tips of the toes. In this text, "thigh" will be used to refer to the region between the knee and the hip, while "lower leg" will be used to refer to the region between the knee and the ankle. Each lower limb consists of 30 bones, the majority of which (26 in total) are located in the foot and ankle. The bones of the thigh and lower leg are the femur, patella, tibia, and fibula.

The femur articulates proximally with the pelvis at the hip and distally with the tibia and patella at the knee. The tibia articulates with the femur, patella, and fibula proximally at the knee and with the fibula and talus distally at the ankle, and is connected to the fibula throughout by an interosseous membrane.

Blood supply to the leg stems primarily from the external iliac artery, which becomes the femoral artery after it passes the inguinal ligament at the hip, and the obturator artery. The lumbar plexus is the source of the majority of nerve supply to the lower extremity and arises from the first four lumbar nerves with some contribution from the subcostal nerve. While a number of peripheral nerves innervate the lower extremities, the sciatic, femoral, and common peroneal nerves are most at risk due to the positions sustained during gaming.

4.1.2   Evaluation

While a lesser degree of understanding of specific gaming mechanics is required for lower extremity assessment, it remains absolutely key for practitioners to be cognizant of the demands of gaming with regard to duration of sitting, frequency of movement, and the "whys" of each. Given the significant amount of time spent sitting, any assessment of lower extremity pathology should also involve an assessment of ergonomics.

4.1.2.1 History Taking

Most players are aware that sitting for long periods of time is not the healthiest of behaviors. Therefore, when taking the history for lower extremity pathology, the tone of the questions asked during the evaluation is just as important as the content.

Location

With regard to the lower extremity, it is important to differentiate deep from superficial pain in order to most accurately identify the structures involved. Deep pain may be more difficult to localize, whereas superficial pain can often be pinpointed with only one finger.

Onset

A player may not notice pain until at the end of a gaming session or when pain becomes significant enough to require a break. Often, pain is normalized and accepted as an expected consequence of prolonged sitting. Recent changes in intensity, duration, or frequency of play, modifications to a player's gaming setup, and non-gaming activities should also be considered.

Palliation and Provocation

Does pain begin as soon as a player sits down, or does it worsen over time? Does pain occur with any other activities? Do transfers, such as sitting to standing or vice versa, cause more pain, or does a change of position relieve it?

Quality

"Burning" is a descriptor most commonly associated with nerve pain, but may also be applied to tendon pain. "Electric" and "radiating" are slightly clearer indicators of nerve involvement, although with prolonged nerve irritation, players may experience deep, achy, or cramping pain as well as fatigue and heaviness. Postural muscle injuries may be described as "achy," "stiff," or "sore," while sequelae in the more distal joints may be sharper, for example, sharp lateral knee pain with iliotibial (IT) band syndrome.

Radiation

When assessing for potential nerve involvement, it is important to consider both dermatomal (Fig. 3.3) and peripheral nerve (Fig. 4.1) distributions. Radiation that follows dermatomal lines may be related to spinal nerve pathology. Pain that remains local without radiation is less likely to be nerve-related and more likely to involve musculotendinous structures.

Esports History

While the specific mechanics of a player's game may not be relevant, an understanding of a player's schedule with regard to daily practice, tournaments, and any streaming obligations will give a clearer picture of their demands.

4.1.2.2 Physical Examination

Inspection

Subtle clues and diagnostic details can be glimmered from simple inspection. The area should be completely exposed to allow for thorough evaluation. Inspection can reveal things such as swelling, erythema, and deformity.

Palpation

Examiners should take care to move from areas of decreased to increased tenderness. Starting in an area of maximal symptoms may lead to guarding and hamper further investigation. Palpation is useful for identifying inflammation, muscle tension, and recreating pain.

Range of Motion

Both active and passive range of motion (ROM) should be assessed to differentiate between musculotendinous and non-musculotendinous injuries, as well as to identify compensations or functional limitations resulting from the disorder.

Sensory Examination

As stated above, an understanding of dermatomal versus peripheral distributions is valuable for differentiating lumbar and lower extremity pathologies.

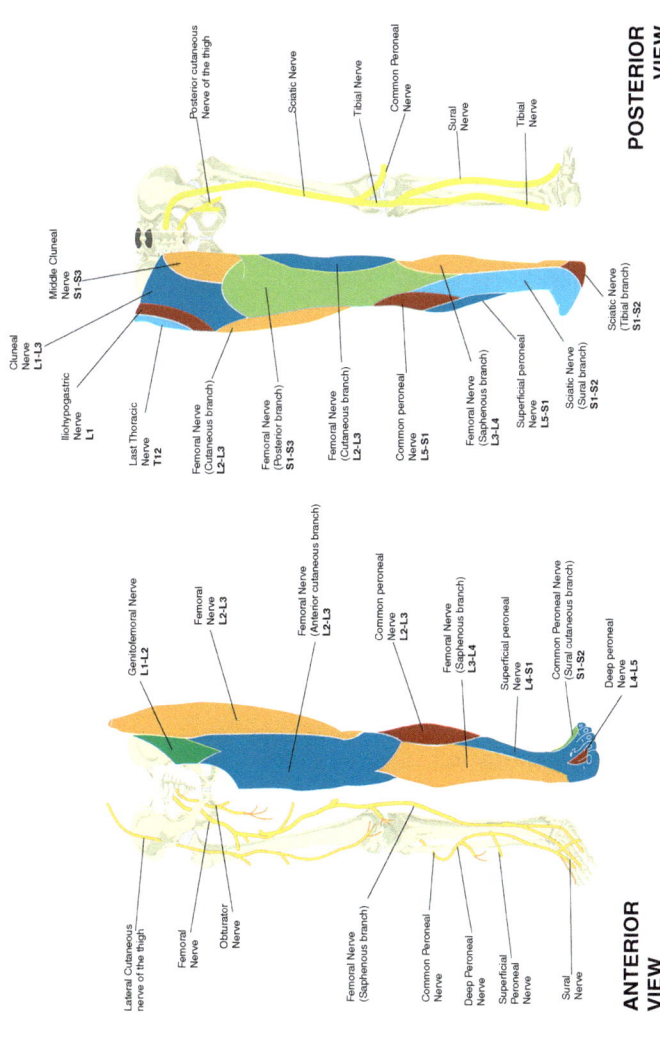

Fig. 4.1 Peripheral sensory nerves of the lower extremity and their corresponding areas of innervation

Motor Examination

Manual muscle testing is useful not only for identifying muscular imbalances, but also for differentiating underlying causes. Manual muscle testing should always be performed bilaterally, even if symptoms are only unilateral, in order to establish a baseline level of strength.

Reflex Examination

Deep tendon reflexes can be elicited by briskly tapping the tendon of a partially stretched muscle. A vital part of the neurological examination, abnormal findings can be used to help pinpoint potential injury levels.

4.1.3 Treatment

4.1.3.1 Therapeutic Modalities

Thermal modalities are commonly utilized to address pain as they are readily accessible in a home treatment setting. Ice is primarily used by the general public to address pain related to inflammation, while heat is used to address pain related to muscle tightness.

While evidence is mixed on the use of transcutaneous electrical nerve stimulation for chronic or neuropathic pain [1], there is tentative evidence to suggest that it is an appropriate intervention for acute pain [2].

4.1.3.2 Rehabilitation

Conservative treatment should be pursued extensively prior to more aggressive interventions such as surgery. Referral to a rehabilitation professional such as a physical therapist allows for an individualized plan of care designed to address the patient's specific deficits.

4.1.3.3 Pharmacology

Topical and oral non-steroidal anti-inflammatory medications (NSAIDs) may provide pain relief, particularly in the acute phases of injury when inflammation is maximal. However, long-term usage can cause gastrointestinal and kidney issues. For neuropathic conditions, anticonvulsant or antidepressant may be more effective.

4.1.3.4 Interventions

On the spectrum between conservative rehabilitation measures and surgical intervention, treatments such as corticosteroid injections, regenerative medicine injections, nerve blocks, and radio-frequency ablation fall somewhere in the middle. Current best practice guidelines recommend use of ultrasound guidance for injections and nerve blocks. In the long term, repeated steroid injections may damage healthy tissues and cause degeneration of cartilaginous structures. Therefore, regenerative medicine injections such a prolotherapy or platelet-rich plasma (PRP) are being considered more often.

4.2   Deep Vein Thrombosis

DVT, Venous Thromboembolism.

4.2.1   Overview

Deep vein thromboses (DVTs) have historically been correlated with periods of prolonged immobility due to debility or postsurgical states. Gaming populations are at elevated risk for this condition as a result of long gameplay sessions. Chang et al. reported in 2013 on a case of deep vein thrombosis in a gamer, and several other cases of gaming DVTs have been identified [3]. Most notably, Geoff Robinson, one of the founding figures of Starcraft, was diagnosed with a DVT and later died of a pulmonary embolism.

4.2.2   Pathogenesis

Thromboses can occur in any vein but the risks of prolonged sitting primarily impact those of the lower extremity. The most commonly affected veins are the femoral, popliteal, posterior tibial, and peroneal veins [4]. Prolonged immobility decreases the pumping action of the muscles of the lower extremities, which stagnates venous return. This muscle action is necessary due to the lower pressure gradient of the veins in the lower extremities.

DVTs can occur in both healthy and unhealthy individuals who sit for prolonged periods, but there are a number of factors which elevate an individual's risk, including:

- Smoking
- Dehydration
- Long air travel
- Blood clotting disorders
- Obesity
- Recent injury/surgery to the region
- Pregnancy
- Use of certain oral contraceptives
- Use of certain hormone replacement therapies
- Cancer
- Heart failure
- Acute inflammatory bowel diseases

4.2.3   Presentation

Unilateral DVTs are significantly more common than bilateral diagnoses. Patients may present with pain, a sensation of pressure, redness, inflammation, warmth near the site of thrombosis, coolness distal to the site of the thrombosis, and fatigue.

Pulmonary Embolism Warning Signs
A pulmonary embolism (PE) is a serious complication of a DVT that occurs when the clot migrates to vessels of the lungs. Warning signs of a PE include:

- Sudden shortness of breath without exertion
- Sudden increased heart rate without exertion
- Pain/pressure in chest, especially with deep breaths
- Hemoptysis
- Dizziness/fainting

4.2.4 Diagnosis

Initial screening is often performed according to the Wells Criteria [5, 6]. This criteria tallies susceptibilities, signs, and symptoms and is shown in Table 4.1. The Wells tool is validated for use in outpatient and trauma patients. It cannot be used to screen for upper extremity DVT.

Depending on availability of testing and suspected thrombosis location, duplex ultrasonography, compression ultrasonography, or color Doppler imaging may be used. In addition to venous

Table 4.1 Wells clinical decision tool [5, 6]

Criteria	Points
Active cancer: ongoing treatment, within previous 6 months, or palliative	1
Paralysis, paresis, or recent immobilization of LE	1
Recently bedridden for >3 days or major surgery within 4 weeks	1
Localized tenderness along deep venous system distribution assessed by firm palpation in posterior calf, popliteal space, and along femoral vein in anterior thigh and groin	1
Entire LE swelling	1
Calf swelling >3 cm compared to asymptomatic LE, measured 10 cm below tibial tuberosity	1
Pitting edema	1
Collateral non varicose superficial veins	1
Alternative diagnosis as likely or greater than that of proximal DVT (cellulitis, calf strain, Baker cyst, postoperative swelling)	−2

Tally total points. The probability of a patient having a DVT is:
0: low
1–2: moderate
>3: high

ultrasound, a D-dimer test may be conducted. Given the test's high negative likelihood ratio, it is best used to rule out DVT in patients with low probability per Wells criteria.

Contrast venography is considered the most accurate "gold standard" test for diagnosing blood clots. However, given the invasiveness of this procedure and the reliability of other tests, diagnosis is usually made with a combination of ultrasonography and D-dimer blood tests [4].

4.2.5   Treatment

4.2.5.1 Prevention
In many cases, and particularly in the relatively young and healthy gaming population, preventive measures significantly reduce the incidence of DVTs and the subsequent need for intervention.

Frequent movement is the lowest effort, easiest-to-implement preventive feature. In gamers, this takes the form of not only regular exercise but also regular breaks during gameplay [3, 7]. For individuals at elevated risk, use of compression stockings, pneumatic compression sleeves, or long-term anticoagulants may be used.

4.2.5.2 Intervention
Anticoagulants are the primary interventional treatment for acute DVT. Anticoagulants may be injected (e.g., unfractionated or low molecular weight heparin, enoxaparin) or taken orally (e.g., warfarin, apixaban). After initial acute treatment, patients are usually placed on a maintenance course of warfarin or other Vitamin K inhibitor [8].

Thrombolytics, or "clot busters," are sometimes used to treat more extensive thromboses. They are associated with both improved outcomes and increased risk of serious bleeding complications [9].

In individuals for whom anticoagulant therapy is contraindicated, an inferior vena cava (IVC) filter may be placed to mitigate risk of pulmonary embolism [10].

4.3   Lower Crossed Syndrome

Unterkreuz syndrome

4.3.1   Overview

Lower crossed syndrome refers to a pattern of muscle imbalances in the lower trunk and proximal lower extremities. It is important to note that imbalances in and of themselves may not be pathological, but rather may lead to pain or functional deficits.

4.3.2   Pathogenesis

Lower crossed syndrome is characterized by weakened rectus abdominis, obliques, and gluteal muscles with tightened erector spinae, multifidi, quadratus lumborum, latissimus dorsi, iliopsoas, and tensor fascia latae [11, 12]. Hamstrings may also be tight due to increased compensatory activity.

This condition is associated with prolonged periods of sitting. Sitting with the thighs flexed at the hip joint results in adaptive facilitation and tightening of the hip flexors; maintaining forward lean requires isometric contraction of the low back extensor musculature resulting in the same. Furthermore, decreased functional usage of the anterior abdominal wall and gluteal muscles result in adaptive inhibition of these muscles.

4.3.3   Presentation

Lower crossed syndrome is often identified secondary to complaints of low back, hip, and/or knee pain. As a result of the muscle imbalances described above, patients will present with anterior pelvic tilt and lumbar hyperlordosis on observation. This results in a posterior shift of the center of mass, often compensated for with increased thoracic kyphosis (and, potentially with corresponding upper crossed syndrome). Additional compensatory movements include lateral lumbar shift, hip external rotation, and knee hyperextension.

4.3.4 Diagnosis

Diagnosis for lower crossed syndrome is primarily achieved through clinical examination. Postural analysis is key to identification of lower crossed syndrome. Patients should be observed both in erect standing and during ambulation for the above postural abnormalities.

Manual muscle testing of the hip extensors and hip abductors will assist with identification of compensatory mechanisms, particularly increased paraspinal activity to compensate for decreased gluteus maximus strength and increased tensor fascia latae/iliopsoas activity to compensate for decreased gluteus medius strength. This results in hip lateral rotation and flexion with abduction testing.

Clinical tests for lower crossed syndrome are shown in Table 4.2. The Thomas test should be used to assess hip flexor flexibility while a straight leg raise assessment should be used to assess hamstring flexibility. The Trendelenburg test should also be used to assess glute function and hip stability.

4.3.5 Treatment

Treatment for lower crossed syndrome addresses two fundamental categories. Effective strategies must not only directly address muscle imbalances, but also subsequent lifestyle changes.

Generally, muscles identified as inhibited should be strengthened and muscles identified as overly facilitated should be inhibited. Stretching of tight muscles without strengthening of weakened muscles will result in minimal, if any, change. Further, passive stretching alone is less effective than active stretching to increase ROM in the lower extremity [13].

Stretching exercises should be coupled with core stabilization exercises, strengthening of the gluteal muscles, and propriocep-

Table 4.2 Clinical tests for lower crossed syndrome

Clinical test	Description
Thomas test	Patient supine. Bring both legs into hip and knee flexion, drawing the knee to the chest until the patient achieves neutral pelvic positioning. Passively lower the affected leg into extension until anterior pelvic tilt occurs, then assess whether patient is able to achieve hip extension or remains flexed.
Straight leg raise	Patient supine. Keep non-testing leg straight and in contact with table. Passively elevate testing leg, maintaining full knee extension, until significant resistance is met, non-testing begins to lift off of table, or knee begins to flex. Measure degree of hip flexion. This test should not be confused with a Straight Leg Raise Test for nerve root sensitivity (Lasègue's sign).
Trendelenburg (stance)	Patient stands on one leg. Observe pelvic positioning. Test is positive for weakness on stance leg if patient's pelvis is higher on the stance leg than on the non-stance leg (uncompensated) OR if patient's pelvis is lower on the stance leg than on non-stance leg (compensated).

tive and neuromuscular re-education. This is best accomplished with the assistance of a trained physical therapist.

> **Passive Versus Active Stretching**
> Active stretching involves the contraction of agonist muscles to stretch antagonist muscles. Passive stretching relies on an external force to create a stretch, such as the use of a stretching strap or assistance from a partner.

4.4   Proximal Hamstring Tendinopathy

4.4.1   Overview

Most proximal or insertional hamstring tendinopathy injuries develop as a result of running and activities involving rapid deceleration and sharp pivots. However, they may also develop as a result of prolonged periods of sitting.

4.4.2 Pathogenesis

The most common cause of proximal hamstring tendinopathy is repetitive hamstring contraction while the hip is flexed, resulting in higher tensile and compressive loads at the insertion of the hamstring. Other causes of hamstring tendinopathy include excessive static stretching and prolonged sitting [14].

A number of factors elevate an individual's risk for hamstring tendinopathy, including joint laxity, decreased flexibility, tight/weak hamstrings and quadriceps, poor lumbopelvic/core stability, and poor proprioception.

4.4.3 Presentation

Patients will present with a gradual onset of deep buttock and posterior thigh pain that is provoked with long periods of sitting, deep hip flexion, and stretching. As with other tendon injuries, in the acute phase, this presents as worse at onset of activity, improving with some degree of warm-up, and then once again worsening with increased activity. Patients may experience weakness as a result of pain-related muscle inhibition.

Patients are unlikely to experience pain with walking, standing, or lying. Prolonged sitting and repetitive motions requiring a higher degree of loading, like running, are likely to increase pain.

4.4.4 Diagnosis

A number of pain provocation clinical tests (Table 4.3) have been developed to aid the clinician in making an accurate diagnosis of proximal hamstring tendinopathy, including the bent-knee stretch test and the Puranen-Orava test. These tests have high sensitivity and specificity per reliability and validity testing. Palpation of the ischial tuberosity can also contribute to clinical diagnosis of proximal hamstring tendinopathy [15, 16].

Table 4.3 Clinical tests for hamstring tendinopathy

Clinical test	Description
Bent-knee stretch test	Patient supine. Passively bring testing leg into maximal hip and knee flexion. Maintain hip flexion while extending knee passively. A positive test is indicated by posterior thigh pain that worsens as knee is further extended
Puranen-Orava test	Patient stands next to table or bench, raises leg into hip and knee flexion, and places heel of testing leg on that surface. Patient then straightens knee and reaches toward toe. A positive test is indicated by posterior thigh pain that worsens as knee is further extended.

Differential Diagnosis
The differential diagnosis for hamstring tendinopathy includes referred lumbar spinal pain, piriformis syndrome, chronic compartment syndrome of the posterior thigh, and ischiofemoral impingement.

When the diagnosis is unclear, musculoskeletal ultrasound or Magnetic Resonance Imaging (MRI) can show tendon thickening, tearing, and inflammation.

4.4.5   Treatment

Principles of progressive loading are an important component of the treatment plan for proximal hamstring tendinopathy. Patients should begin with isometric hamstring loading in a neutral hip position, followed by progression to isotonic loading in a minimally flexed position, and finally isotonic loading in 70–90° of hip flexion. In the early phase of recovery, hamstring stretching, trunk flexion, and repeated lifting should be **avoided** [17, 18].

It is important to note that while passive treatments including modalities and soft tissue mobilization may be used to alleviate pain, they will not improve load capacity and should only be used to complement or supplement more active interventions [19].

Load modification and ergonomic changes are also key to recovery from tendinopathy. Patients who sit for prolonged periods may benefit from the use of a shaped cushion to offload the irritated area.

Shaped Cushions for Hamstring Tendinopathy
For proximal hamstring tendinopathy, a cushion can be used to offload the proximal hamstring tendon. This can either be a pillow with additional bulk in the front, putting more pressure on the hamstring muscle belly, or a shaped ergonomic pillow that is contoured to the shape of the thighs and buttocks.

Research is mixed on the value and efficacy of NSAIDs with regard to tendon injuries. While NSAIDs can decrease pain and inflammation, they may also inhibit tendon healing.

When conservative treatment is insufficient, a corticosteroid injection into the soft tissues surrounding the tendon may be beneficial with regard to pain and inflammation. This has been shown to be more effective in patients with less severe tendon thickening [20]. However, corticosteroid injections can result in weakening of load-bearing tendons and are not a long-term solution; they are most beneficial when used in conjunction with physical therapy for progressive loading. Injection of platelet-rich plasma or prolotherapy has also been proposed as a potential alternative to corticosteroid injections to promote tissue healing; however, there is insufficient evidence to support their widespread use at this time.

4.5   Piriformis Syndrome

Extra-spinal sciatica, deep gluteal syndrome, wallet neuritis.

4.5.1   Overview

Piriformis syndrome is a musculoskeletal condition in which peripheral branches of the sciatic nerves are irritated by an abnormal condition of the piriformis muscle.

4.5.2 Pathogenesis

The most common anatomical relationship between the piriformis and sciatic nerve involves the sciatic nerve exiting the greater sciatic foramen along the inferior surface of the piriformis. Documented anatomical variations from this course include the sciatic nerve passing through the piriformis, superiorly to the piriformis, or the tibial branch splitting from the main portion of the sciatic nerve and passing either inferiorly or superiorly to the piriformis separately from that main branch. It was previously thought that these variations may predispose to a higher risk of piriformis syndrome. However, research has not found a significant difference in the prevalence of anomalous anatomical variations in patients with piriformis syndrome relative to the prevalence in the uninjured population [21].

Despite this shift in understanding, piriformis syndrome in which an anatomical variation of the sciatic nerve is identified is referred to as primary piriformis syndrome. Secondary piriformis syndrome is the result of some external cause like muscle spasms secondary to lumbar or sacroiliac pathologies, altered biomechanics of the low back and pelvic regions, microtrauma from direct compression (i.e., "wallet neuritis") or overuse, or macrotrauma to the buttocks resulting in soft tissue inflammation .

Rarer causes of piriformis syndrome may include bursitis of the piriformis, colorectal carcinoma, episacroiliac lipoma, Klippel-Trenaunay syndrome, abscess or hematoma, neoplasms in the area of the infrapiriform foramen, irritation following intragluteal injection, and myositis ossificans of the piriformis muscle.

Piriformis syndrome is more common in women due to the wider angle of the quadratus femoris in the pelvic girdle.

4.5.3 Presentation

Patients often complain of a pressure like pain in the buttocks. This may radiate down the posterior thigh with resulting paresthesia and pain-related inhibition may be present. Patients frequently report irritation with prolonged sitting or walking, squatting, and positions that increase the tension of the piriformis muscle, such as hip adduction and internal rotation.

Patients may also demonstrate a "splayfoot sign" with hip external rotation during standing, walking, or lying in supine [22].

4.5.4 Diagnosis

Piriformis syndrome may be diagnosed via clinical testing or with diagnostic injections.

4.5.4.1 Physical Examination

Clinical testing of piriformis syndrome should include palpation of the greater sciatic notch and of the piriformis muscle belly. Deep palpation of the retro-trochanteric region may elicit leg numbness and an exacerbation of tightness [23]. With most cases, there is no loss of deep tendon reflexes or weakness in a myotomal pattern.

A number of clinical assessments (Table 4.4) are also valuable for identifying piriformis syndrome and differentiating it from other, similar conditions.

Differential Diagnosis
Differential diagnosis of piriformis syndrome includes trochanteric bursitis, lumbosacral radiculopathies or facet syndromes, sacroiliac pathologies, lumbar spinal stenosis, referred pain from pelvic visceral malignancies or diseases of the appendix and renal system, and intra-articular hip pathologies.

Beatty's maneuver in particular is useful for distinguishing between piriformis syndrome and lumbar discogenic pain, as patients with piriformis syndrome will experience deep buttock pain while patients with lumbar discogenic issues will experience back and leg pain [24].

Table 4.4 Clinical tests for piriformis syndrome

Clinical test	Description
Pace's sign	Position patient in sitting with testing leg in abduction and external rotation, then apply resistance. A positive result is indicated by pain with resisted abduction and external rotation.
Straight leg raise test	Patient supine. Passively raise testing leg. A positive result is indicated by recreation of radiating LE pain.
Freiberg sign	Patient supine. Passively bring leg into maximal internal hip rotation. A positive result is indicated by recreation of radiating LE pain.
FADIR test	Position patient in sidelying with testing leg on top. Passively bring leg into 90 degrees of hip flexion, adduction, and internal rotation. A positive result is indicated by pain in the gluteal region.
Beatty's maneuver	Position patient in sidelying with testing leg on top. Passively bring leg into 90 degrees of hip flexion. Instruct patient to perform abduction, and resist patient's attempt. A positive result is indicated by pain in the buttock region.

4.5.4.2 Imaging and Diagnostics

The role of further diagnostics is limited, as imaging is more useful for ruling out other conditions. Ultrasound-guided injections may be used for therapeutic as well as diagnostic purposes.

4.5.5 Treatment

Conservative treatment methods are the mainstay of effective treatment [25]. Pharmacological agents can be utilized for pain control, such as NSAIDs, muscle relaxants, and neuropathic pain medications. When pain is appropriately managed, physical therapy and lifestyle modifications can be instituted to promote recovery. Physical therapy should include strengthening of the hip extensors, abductors, and external rotators; soft tissue mobilizations; and piriformis stretching. Lifestyle modifications may include increasing frequency of standing/walking breaks while sitting every 20 min, incorporating daily stretching, and making stops during long drives to stand and change position.

Ultrasound-guided injections of the piriformis with anesthetics, corticosteroid, or chemodenervation may address cases refractory to conservative management.

Surgical interventions such as tenotomy of the piriformis tendon or release of the internal obturator muscle should only be considered with intractable, disabling symptoms for which a trial of conservative management has failed. Additional indications for surgical intervention include the presence of an abscess, neoplasm, hematoma, or painful vascular compression from gluteal varicosity.

4.6   Sacroiliac Joint Pathology

SIJ dysfunction, Sacroiliitis.

4.6.1   Overview

Sacroiliac (SI) joint pathologies result in back pain that may be misdiagnosed as radicular lumbar pain and subsequently mistreated by clinicians. This condition is remarkably common, and contributes to 10–27% of low back pain cases [26].

4.6.2   Pathogenesis

The primary function of the sacroiliac joints is load transfer between the spine and lower extremities, which requires a balance of mobility and stability mediated both passively by ligamentous structures and actively by muscular attachments on the sacrum and innominate bones. Dysfunction of any of these structures can result in SIJ pathology.

The most straightforward causes of sacroiliac joint dysfunction result from direct trauma to the region, as in a motor vehicle accident, and the release of relaxin during pregnancy resulting in increased ligamentous laxity.

SI joint dysfunction is more common in obese individuals and individuals who lead sedentary lifestyles. This likely reflects a number of factors including postural strain on the passive ligamentous structures supporting this region and decreased active support secondary to decreased muscular strength and endurance.

4.6.3 Presentation

Symptoms of SI joint dysfunction are very similar to symptoms of other types of low back pain, which may confound diagnosis. In fact, "low back pain" is the most commonly reported symptom associated with SI joint dysfunction. This pain may be localized to the posterior aspect of the joint or refer down the posterior thigh, usually not past the knee. Pain will worsen with mechanical stress of the SI joint, as during forward trunk flexion or stair ascent/descent.

4.6.4 Diagnosis

Given the similarity in symptoms between this pathology and other types of low back pain, any diagnosis of SI joint dysfunction must include mechanisms to rule out other potential causes.

4.6.4.1 Physical Examination

Differential Diagnosis
The differential diagnoses for SI joint pathology includes radicular pain, piriformis syndrome, ankylosing spondylitis, lumbosacral facet syndrome, spondyloarthropathy, and trochanteric bursitis.

Most diagnoses are made with a combination of ruling out other back pain sources and ruling in SI joint dysfunction using provocative clinical tests [27]. No single test has a particularly high sensitivity or specificity, and are subsequently used in

Table 4.5 Clinical tests for SI joint dysfunction

Clinical test	Description
Gaenslen test	Position patient in supine with testing leg at edge of the table, almost off the side. Patient holds non-testing leg in hip and knee flexion. Passively abduct testing leg just enough to lower into hip extension with knee flexion off the side of the table. Apply hyperextension overpressure to testing leg and flexion overpressure to non-testing leg. A positive test is indicated by reproduction of the patient's pain.
Sacral thrust	Patient prone. Apply anterior pressure to center of sacrum to create shear force across both SI joints. A positive test is indicated by reproduction of pain in sacroiliac region.
SI joint compression test	Position patient in sidelying. Apply downward pressure on superior iliac crest, directing force at opposite iliac crest. A positive test is indicated by reproduction of pain in sacroiliac region.
SI joint distraction test	Patient supine. Apply posterolateral pressure to bilateral anterior superior iliac spine. A positive test is indicated by reproduction of pain.
FABER test	Patient supine. Place patient in "Fig. 4" position with hip in flexion and abduction, knee in flexion, and lateral ankle resting on opposite thigh proximal to the knee. Stabilize the opposite side of the pelvis at the anterior superior iliac spine, then apply a posterior force to the knee of the testing leg. A positive test is indicated by reproduction of pain or limited range of motion relative to the contralateral leg.
Yeoman test	Patient prone. Passive flex the knee of the leg to be tested to 90 degrees. Stabilize the ipsilateral pelvis and passively extend the hip of the testing leg. A positive test is indicated by pain in the SI joint.

combination with others. As such, clinicians should use at least three tests shown in Table 4.5 to make an accurate diagnosis [28].

4.6.4.2 Imaging

Computerized tomography (CT) and MRI are useful primarily as "rule-out" diagnostic tools to identify arthritis, multiple myeloma, stenosis, bursitis, fracture, herniation, or tendinopathy. As with piriformis syndrome, ultrasound-guided injection is valuable both as a diagnostic and therapeutic tool, particularly in patients with isolated and localized pain or patients with positive results on a cluster of clinical tests [29, 30].

4.6.5   Treatment

Best outcomes in the treatment of SI joint dysfunction result from a multidisciplinary care model. With physical therapy, treatment should involve reducing inflammation if present, addressing hypomobility with joint mobilization/manipulation, and addressing hypermobility or instability with core stabilization and motor control exercises. Patients should also receive education in postural and ergonomic modifications [31].

In patients for whom chronic low back pain has developed as a result of SI joint dysfunction, ablation of the nociceptive nerve fibers may be appropriate [32].

4.7   Compressive Neuropathies of the Lower Extremity

4.7.1   General

4.7.1.1 Overview

While compressive neuropathies of the upper extremity, such as carpal tunnel syndrome or radial tunnel syndrome, are more common and certainly more well-known in the general population, compressive neuropathies of the lower extremity remain an important consideration for gaming populations. In this section, we explore the three nerves most at risk in the esports population.

4.7.1.2 Pathogenesis

Nerve entrapment most commonly occurs in anatomical regions where the nerve passes by or through another structure, such as a fascial opening, a bony groove or fissure, or a muscle belly. Pressures as low as 20 mm Hg are enough to affect signal transmission along a nerve, with higher pressures resulting in more significant blocks to nerve conduction. As a general rule, the longer and more significant the compression, the longer the recovery.

Nerve entrapments may be broadly divided into three stages [33].

- Stage I: Intermittent paresthesias and sensory deficits, most commonly at night
- Stage II: Dexterity and endurance are impacted and symptoms become consistent
- Stage III: Morphological changes, such as segmental demyelination and increased edema, occur

4.7.1.3 Diagnosis

A thorough history taking is essential, including knowledge of a player's preferred postures and points of potential compression resulting from their gaming ergonomics. As emphasized previously, knowledge of dermatomal and peripheral nerve distributions is key to identifying the origin of nerve-related pathology.

Ultrasonography, electrophysiological testing, and advanced imaging may also be of diagnostic importance in severe or unclear cases [34, 35].

4.7.1.4 Treatment

Appropriate interventions for these conditions fall into two categories: symptomatic care and preventive care. Symptomatic care focuses on mitigating pain and can include therapeutic exercise, bracing, manual therapy, injections, and NSAIDs or neuropathic pain medications. These should be designed to address a player's specific symptoms. Preventive care involves first identifying the factors originally leading to compression, such as posture, type or size of chair, provoking activities, or even restrictive clothing. Once provocations have been determined, interventions to remove them can be instituted. This may involve ergonomic changes or activity modification.

4.7.2 Common Peroneal Nerve

4.7.2.1 Overview

Peroneal neuropathy is the most common lower extremity compressive neuropathy [36]. The common peroneal nerve originates centrally from fibers of the L4-S1 nerve roots and branches peripherally off of the sciatic nerve above the popliteal fossa, providing motor innervation to ankle everters, ankle dorsiflexors, and toe dorsiflexors and providing sensory innervation to the lateral lower leg and the dorsum of the foot. It is vulnerable to compression due to its positioning against the fibular head.

Risk factors for this condition include positions of prolonged knee flexion, positions involving prolonged leg crossing, and low bodyweight [37].

> **Fibular Versus Peroneal**
> A long-standing debate between anatomists and clinicians, the two terms refer to identical structures.

4.7.2.2 Presentation

The characteristic hallmark of this compressive neuropathy is foot drop. Prior to this development, players may complain of numbness over the lateral lower leg and dorsum of the foot, or paresthesia radiating down the sensory distribution.

4.7.2.3 Diagnosis

Patients should be questioned about potential risk factors, such a propensity to cross the legs. On examination of a patient's gait, foot drop may be noticed. Manual muscle testing can reveal weakness in the muscles innervation by the common peroneal nerve, as well as numbness in the sensory distribution. Abnormal deep tendon reflexes of the quadriceps or Achilles tendons support a more proximal diagnosis.

Nerve conduction testing and needle electromyography are appropriate diagnostic modalities and may also provide insight into the severity of injury.

> **Differential Diagnosis**
> Foot drop may also occur with sciatic nerve injury, lumbosacral nerve injury, or L4-S1 radiculopathy.

4.7.2.4 Treatment

As with other lower extremity compressive neuropathies, conservative management including physical therapy, activity, and ergonomic modification, and bracing are appropriate interventions. Surgical intervention is rarely required and generally not recommended.

4.7.3 Sciatic Nerve

4.7.3.1 Overview

The sciatic nerve is the largest nerve in the human body. It originates centrally from fibers of the L4-S3 nerve routes. It passes through the pelvis and into the gluteal region at the greater sciatic foramen and exits either under, through, or around the piriformis muscle. From there, it courses between the gluteus maximus and the quadratus femoris, and runs between the hamstrings and the adductor magnus until it divides into the common peroneal and tibial nerves just above the popliteal fossa.

Compression may result from prolonged sitting or pressure, female sex, hamstring injury, or piriformis hypertrophy [23, 38, 39].

> **Wallet Neuritis**
> Individuals who consistently wear their wallet in their rear pocket on the same side and do not remove it prior to sitting may develop direct sciatic nerve irritation.

4.7.3.2 Presentation

Players may complain of numbness, tingling, and pain in the buttock and posterior-lateral leg. With prolonged compression, radiation may occur as far as the knee.

4.7.3.3 Diagnosis

As with other peripheral neuropathies, this condition must be differentiated from lumbar radiculopathies and facet arthropathies. Clinical diagnosis should, therefore, include a neurological examination of the lower limb, palpation at potential sites of entrapment for provocation, and use of the straight leg raise test to elicit LaSegue's sign. It is important to note that while this test has high sensitivity, it has low specificity [40]. LaSegue's sign alone is not sufficient for a diagnosis of sciatic nerve entrapment.

Clinical examination may be combined with electrodiagnostic studies, MRI, or diagnostic injection.

4.7.3.4 Treatment

Treatment is dependent on the location of the site of entrapment. Conservative interventions including therapeutic exercise, modalities, and soft tissue or joint mobilization form the first line of defense. Ultrasound- or fluoroscopic-guided injection may be performed for therapeutic as well as for diagnostic purposes. In cases occurring as a result of hip fracture or compartment syndrome, or in patients who have not experienced significant improvement following conservative interventions, surgical release of the nerve may be appropriate [41].

4.7.4 Femoral Nerve

4.7.4.1 Overview

Femoral compressive neuropathy is less common than either sciatic or peroneal entrapments and most commonly occurs secondary to surgery [42]. The femoral nerve is derived centrally from the L2-L4 nerve roots. It passes under the inguinal ligament to enter the anterior thigh and immediately divides into anterior and lateral divisions to provide sensory and motor innervation to the anterior thigh.

4.7.4.2 Presentation

The primary symptom of femoral nerve entrapment is weakness of the quadriceps muscle. Players with compressive neuropathy occurring *above* the inguinal ligament will present with hip flexor weakness, while players with compressive neuropathy occurring *below* the inguinal ligament will not.

4.7.4.3 Diagnosis

When examining players for this condition, consider if their motor and sensory deficits match the sensory distribution of the femoral nerve (anterior and medial thigh sensation) or if other nerve distributions are involved (e.g., lateral thigh sensation from the obturator nerve). Severe injury may result in patellar tendon reflex deficits. The modified Thomas Test, with combined hip extension and knee flexion, is likely to recreate symptoms [43]. To perform this test, position the patient in supine with hips at the very end of the table. The patient should hold the non-testing leg in maximal knee and hip flexion, allowing the testing leg to hang freely. This test is primarily used to assess deficits in the quadriceps, rectus femoris, psoas, or tensor fascia lata muscles, but may also result in recreation of pain in patients with femoral nerve entrapment.

Nerve conduction studies are of limited utility for diagnosis of femoral nerve entrapment, as only the portions distal to the inguinal ligament can be assessed via traditional techniques. Ultrasound or MRI may be appropriate when an injury proximal to the inguinal ligament is suspected [44].

4.7.4.4 Treatment

Manual therapy, therapeutic exercise, stretching, ergonomic changes, injections, and education are all appropriate components of a conservative intervention plan [45]. Surgical interventions such as neurolysis or neurectomy should only be considered when symptoms fail to respond well to conservative management.

References

1. Gibson W, Wand BM, Meads C, Catley MJ, O'Connell NE. Transcutaneous electrical nerve stimulation (TENS) for chronic pain – an overview of Cochrane Reviews. Cochrane Database Syst Rev. 2019;2(2):CD011890. https://doi.org/10.1002/14651858.CD011890.pub3.
2. Johnson MI, Paley CA, Howe TE, Sluka KA. Transcutaneous electrical nerve stimulation for acute pain. Cochrane Database Syst Rev. 2015;6(6):CD006142. https://doi.org/10.1002/14651858.CD006142.pub3.
3. Chang HCL, Burbridge H, Wong C. Extensive deep vein thrombosis following prolonged gaming ('gamer's thrombosis'): a case report. J Med Case Rep. 2013;7(1) https://doi.org/10.1186/1752-1947-7-235.
4. Kesieme E, Kesieme C, Jebbin N, Irekpita E, Dongo A. Deep vein thrombosis: a clinical review. J Blood Med. 2011;2:59–69. https://doi.org/10.2147/JBM.S19009.
5. Wells PS, Anderson DR, Bormanis J, Guy F, Mitchell M, Gray L, et al. Value of assessment of pretest probability of deep-vein thrombosis in clinical management. Lancet. 1997;350(9094):1795–8. https://doi.org/10.1016/S0140-6736(97)08140-3.
6. Wells PS, Anderson DR, Rodger M, Forgie M, Kearon C, Dreyer J, et al. Evaluation of D-dimer in the diagnosis of suspected deep-vein thrombosis. N Engl J Med. 2003;349:1227–35. https://doi.org/10.1056/NEJMoa023153.
7. Hillegass E, Puthoff M, Frese EM, Thigpen M, Sobush DC, Auten B. Role of physical therapists in the management of individuals at risk for or diagnosed with venous thromboembolism: evidence-based clinical practice guideline. Phys Ther. 2016;96(2):143–66.
8. Snow V, Qaseem A, Barry P, Rodney Hornbake E, Rodnick JE, Tobolic T, et al. Management of venous thromboembolism: a clinical practice guideline from the American College of Physicians and the American Academy of Family Physicians. Ann Intern Med. 2007;146(3):204–10. https://doi.org/10.7326/0003-4819-146-3-200702060-00149.
9. Watson L, Broderick C, Armon M. Thrombolysis for acute deep vein thrombosis. Cochrane Database Syst Rev. 2016;11(11):CD002783. https://doi.org/10.1002/14651858.CD002783.pub4.
10. Decousus H, Leizorovicz A, Parent F, Page Y, Tardy B, Girard P, et al. A clinical trial of vena caval filters in the prevention of pulmonary embolism in patients with proximal deep-vein thrombosis. N Engl J Med. 1998;338(7):409–15. https://doi.org/10.1056/NEJM199802123380701.
11. Key J. The pelvic crossed syndromes: a reflection of imbalanced function in the myofascial envelope; a further exploration of Janda's work. J Bodyw Mov Ther. 2010;14:299–301. https://doi.org/10.1016/j.jbmt.2010.01.008.

12. Janda V. Muscles and motor control in low back pain: Assessment and management. In: Twomey LT, editor. Physical therapy of the low back. New York/Edinburgh/London: Churchill Livingston; 1987. p. 253–87.

13. Roberts J, Wilson K. Effect of stretching duration on active and passive range of motion in the lower extremity. Br J Sports Med. 1999;33(4):259–63. https://doi.org/10.1136/bjsm.33.4.259.

14. Lempainen L, Sarimo J, Matilla K, Orava S. Proximal hamstring tendinopathy – overview of the problem with emphasis on the surgical treatment. Oper Tech Sports Med. 2009;17:225–8. https://doi.org/10.1053/j.otsm.2009.12.016.

15. Lempainen L, Johansson K, Banke IJ, et al. Expert opinion: diagnosis and treatment of proximal hamstring tendinopathy. Muscles Ligaments Tendons J. 2015;5:23–8.

16. Goom TS, Malliaras P, Reiman MP, Purdam CR. Proximal hamstring tendinopathy: clinical aspects of assessment and management. J Orthop Sports Phys Ther. 2016;46(6):483–93. https://doi.org/10.2519/jospt.2016.5986.

17. Harvey MA, Singh H, Obopilwe E, Charette R, Miller S. Proximal hamstring repair strength: a biomechanical analysis at 3 hip flexion angles. Orthop J Sports Med. 2015;3(4):2325967115576910. https://doi.org/10.1177/2325967115576910.

18. Cook JL, Purdam CR. Is tendon pathology a continuum? A pathology model to explain the clinical presentation of load-induced tendinopathy. Br J Sports Med. 2009;43(6):409–16. https://doi.org/10.1136/bjsm.2008.051193.

19. Guex K, Millet GP. Conceptual framework for strengthening exercises to prevent hamstring strains. Sports Med. 2013;43(12):1207–15. https://doi.org/10.1007/s40279-013-0097-y.

20. Zissen MH, Wallace G, Stevens KJ, Fredericson M, Beaulieu CF. High hamstring tendinopathy: MRI and ultrasound imaging and therapeutic efficacy of percutaneous corticosteroid injection. Am J Roentgenol. 2010;195(4):993–8. https://doi.org/10.2214/AJR.09.3674.

21. Smoll NR. Variations of the piriformis and sciatic nerve with clinical consequence: a review. Clin Anat. 2010;23(1):8–17. https://doi.org/10.1002/ca.20893.

22. Kirschner JS, Foye PM, Cole JL. Piriformis syndrome, diagnosis and treatment. Muscle Nerve. 2009;40(1):10–8. https://doi.org/10.1002/mus.21318.

23. Boyajian-O'Neill LA, McClain RL, Coleman MK, Thomas PP. Diagnosis and management of piriformis syndrome: an osteopathic approach. J Am Osteopath Ass. 2008;108(11):657–64. https://doi.org/10.7556/jaoa.2008.108.11.657.

24. Hopayian K, Song F, Riera R, Sambandan S. The clinical features of the piriformis syndrome: a systematic review. Eur Spine J. 2010;19(12):2095–109. https://doi.org/10.1007/s00586-010-1504-9.

25. Fishman LM, Dombi GW, Michaelsen C, Ringel S, Rozbruch J, Rosner B, Weber C. Piriformis syndrome: diagnosis, treatment, and outcome—a 10-year study. Arch Phys Med. 2002;83(3):295–301. https://doi.org/10.1053/apmr.2002.30622.
26. Raj MA, Varacallo M. Sacroiliac (SI) joint pain. In: StatPearls. StatPearls Publishing. 2019. https://www.ncbi.nlm.nih.gov/books/NBK470299/. Accessed 28 June 2020
27. Zelle BA, Gruen GS, Brown S, George S. Sacroiliac joint dysfunction: evaluation and management. Clin J Pain. 2005;21(5):446–55. https://doi.org/10.1097/01.ajp.0000131413.07468.8e.
28. Broadhurst NA, Bond MJ. Pain provocation tests for the assessment of sacroiliac joint dysfunction. J Spinal Disord. 1998;11(4):341–5. PMID: 9726305
29. D'Orazio F, Gregori LM, Gallucci M. Spine epidural and sacroiliac joints injections—when and how to perform. Eur J Radiol. 2015;84(5):777–82. https://doi.org/10.1016/j.ejrad.2014.05.039.
30. Maigne JY, Aivaliklis A, Pfefer F. Results of sacroiliac joint double block and value of sacroiliac pain provocation tests in 54 patients with low back pain. Spine. 1996;21(16):1889–92. https://doi.org/10.1097/00007632-199608150-00012.
31. Al-Subahi M, Alayat M, Alshehri MA, Helal O, Alhasan H, Alalawi A, et al. The effectiveness of physiotherapy interventions for sacroiliac joint dysfunction: a systematic review. J Phys Ther Sci. 2017;29(9):1689–94. https://doi.org/10.1589/jpts.29.1689.
32. Aydin SM, Gharibo CG, Mehnert M, Stitik TP. The role of radiofrequency ablation for sacroiliac joint pain: a meta-analysis. Am J Phys Med Rehabil. 2010;2(9):842–51. https://doi.org/10.1016/j.pmrj.2010.03.035.
33. Flanigan RM, DiGiovanni BF. Peripheral nerve entrapments of the lower leg, ankle, and foot. Foot Ankle Clin. 2011;16(2):255–74. https://doi.org/10.1016/j.fcl.2011.01.006.
34. Petchprapa CN, Rosenberg ZS, Sconfienza LM, Cavalcanti CF, Vieira RL, Zember JS. MR imaging of entrapment neuropathies of the lower extremity. Part 1. The pelvis and hip. Radiographics. 2010;30(4):983–1000. https://doi.org/10.1148/rg.304095135.
35. Donovan A, Rosenberg ZS, Cavalcanti CF. MR imaging of entrapment neuropathies of the lower extremity. Part 2. The knee, leg, ankle, and foot. Radiographics. 2010;30(4):1001–19. https://doi.org/10.1148/rg.304095188.
36. Bowley MP, Doughty CT. Entrapment neuropathies of the lower extremity. Med Clin N Am. 2018;103(2):371–82. https://doi.org/10.1016/j.mcna.2018.10.013.
37. Cruz-Martinez A, Arpa J, Palau F. Peroneal neuropathy after weight loss. J Peripher Nerv Syst. 2000;5(2):101–5. https://doi.org/10.1046/j.1529-8027.2000.00007.x.

38. Holland NR, Schwartz-Williams L, Blotzer JW. "Toilet seat" sciatic neuropathy. Arch Neurol. 1999;56(1):116. https://doi.org/10.1001/archneur.56.1.116.
39. Wilbourn AJ, Mitsumoto H. Proximal sciatic neuropathies caused by prolonged sitting. Neurology. 1988;38:400.
40. Valat JP, Genevay S, Marty M, Rozenberg S, Koes B. Sciatica. Best Pract Res Clin Rheumol. 2010;24(2):241–52. https://doi.org/10.1016/j.berh.2009.11.005.
41. Kobbe P, Zelle BA, Gruen GS. Case report: recurrent piriformis syndrome after surgical release. Clin Orthop Relat Res. 2008;466(7):1745–8. https://doi.org/10.1007/s11999-008-0151-5.
42. McCrory P, Bell S. Nerve entrapment syndromes as a cause of pain in the hip, groin and buttock. Sports Med. 1999;27:261–74. https://doi.org/10.2165/00007256-199927040-00005.
43. Martin R, Martin HD, Kivlan BR. Nerve entrapment in the hip region: current concepts review. Int J Sports Phys Ther. 2017;12(7):1163–73. https://doi.org/10.26603/ijspt20171163.
44. Gruber H, Peer S, Kovacs P, Marth R, Bodner G. The ultrasonographic appearance of the femoral nerve and cases of iatrogenic impairment. J Ultrasound Med. 2003;22(2) https://doi.org/10.7863/jum.2003.22.2.163.
45. Schmid AB, Nee RJ, Coppieters MW. Reappraising entrapment neuropathies – mechanisms, diagnosis and management. Man Ther. 2013;18:449–57. https://doi.org/10.1016/j.math.2013.07.006.

The Ergonomics of Esports

5

Caitlin McGee

5.1 Neutral Posture

5.1.1 Head and Neck

The head should be placed in a neutral position, with variation expected due to structural differences of the axis (C2). Cervical lordosis develops early on when infants begin to pick up their heads, and should be present in most cases.

Common issues that may arise from a non-neutral head and non-lordotic cervical spine are discussed in depth in Chap. 3.

5.1.2 Trunk and Arms

The natural lordotic curve of the lumbar spine should be supported. Chest should be elevated with mild scapular retraction. Arms should be supported to meet these criteria, in order of priority:

C. McGee (✉)
1HP, Washington, DC, USA

© The Author(s), under exclusive license to Springer Nature Switzerland AG 2021
L. Migliore et al. (eds.), *Handbook of Esports Medicine*,
https://doi.org/10.1007/978-3-030-73610-1_5

1. Wrists are maintained in neutral positioning or mild extension in the coronal plane, and neutral positioning or mild ulnar deviation in the sagittal plane, on mouse and keyboard.
2. Forearms are supported at the level of the navel.
3. Upper arm is supported close to the body, minimizing shoulder abduction.

5.1.3   Lower Extremities

Hips should be maintained in a pelvic neutral positioning. This requires appropriate support for the feet and legs. If the feet are not adequately supported, players tend to compensate with either an anterior or posterior pelvic tilt, as shown in Fig. 5.1. With an anterior pelvic tilt, players compensate with either an accentuated lumbar lordosis or a forward trunk lean with forearm support on the thighs. A posterior pelvic tilt can cause flattening of the lumbar lordosis, and occur in tandem with a backward trunk lean and an excessive thoracic and cervical kyphosis.

With the feet adequately supported, weight is distributed through the thighs as well as through the hips and buttocks, allowing for pelvic neutral positioning.

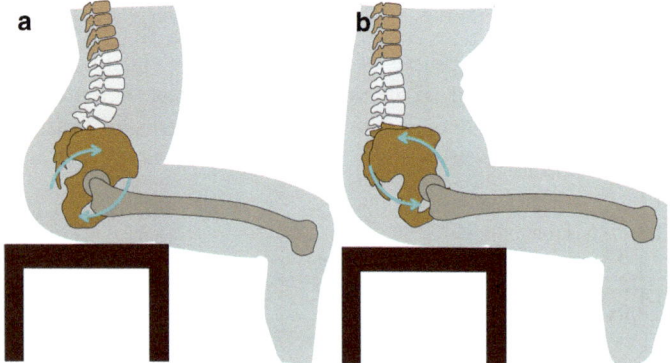

Fig. 5.1 (**a**) Anterior pelvic tilt, accompanied by increased lumbar lordosis. (**b**) Posterior pelvic tilt with flattening of the lumbar lordosis

5.2   Gaming Categories

For the purpose of this section, it is important to define several categories of gaming:

1. PC
2. Console
3. Mobile

> **Virtual Reality Ergonomics**
> This section will not address virtual reality (VR) gaming ergonomics. Depending on the title, VR ergonomics may be similar to the postures and positions trained for in traditional sports, for which there is an abundance of existing literature.

PC games include any games played on a personal computer, most commonly using mouse and keyboard.

Console games include any games played on a gaming console, such as Xbox, Playstation, Gamecube, and Wii. While devices like the Nintendo Gameboy and Nintendo Switch are considered to be consoles, for the purposes of ergonomics we will consider them to be mobile gaming devices.

Mobile games are most commonly played on a smartphone, tablet, or handheld gaming device.

For a more detailed description of the gaming categories and popular titles, Chap. 1 provides an in-depth analysis of the basics of esports.

5.3   Peripherals

5.3.1   Monitor

Monitors should be aligned to minimize cervical flexion, extension, and rotation. In practice, the top of the monitor should be approximately level with the eyebrows. A single monitor should be positioned at the median line of the coronal plane; multiple monitors should be symmetrically distributed about this line [2]. Monitors should be 20–40 inches (50–100 cm) from the eyes.

When monitors are too close, players are more likely to develop convergence-related eyestrain and to assume suboptimal postures, usually involving excessive thoracic kyphosis and posterior pelvic tilt. When monitors are too far, players are more likely to develop eye issues related to squinting, most commonly overuse/strain of the eye muscles and dry eye, as squinting has been shown to reduce blink rate and subsequent lubrication of the surface of the eye [3]. Too-far monitors also put players at risk of increased forward head posture and anterior pelvic tilt/forward trunk lean, reducing external support for the spine and increasing strain on the structures supporting the spine.

5.3.2   Mouse

The optimal size, weight, and sensitivity of a mouse will depend heavily on both the playstyle and the biomechanics of the person using it. However, certain general principles apply across all players.

A mouse that is too tall will provide increased pressure at the distal transverse arch of the palm, promoting a greater degree of wrist extension. Increased wrist extension positions the hand and finger extensors in suboptimal resting length-tension relationships; it also increases pressure in the carpal tunnel. Wrist extension greater than 30 ° increases carpal tunnel pressure by 7%, and extension greater than 45 ° creates a significantly increased risk for musculoskeletal syndromes [4].

The weight of a mouse is also relevant, particularly for players who lift and move their mouse repeatedly as a way to reposition the mouse without repositioning the pointer. This playstyle specifically benefits from a lighter mouse.

Dots Per Inch (DPI) is a measure of mouse sensitivity. When DPI is lower, a player must move the mouse more to accomplish the same in-game movement as someone with a higher DPI. When DPI is higher, smaller volume movements accomplish the same in-game movements, but the increased precision required often results in higher sustained grip forces. No studies have indicated a clear link between higher vs lower DPI and risk of pain or injury.

There are three common mouse grip styles in gaming: palm, claw, and tip as shown in Fig. 5.2. Each of these have their own ergonomic considerations.

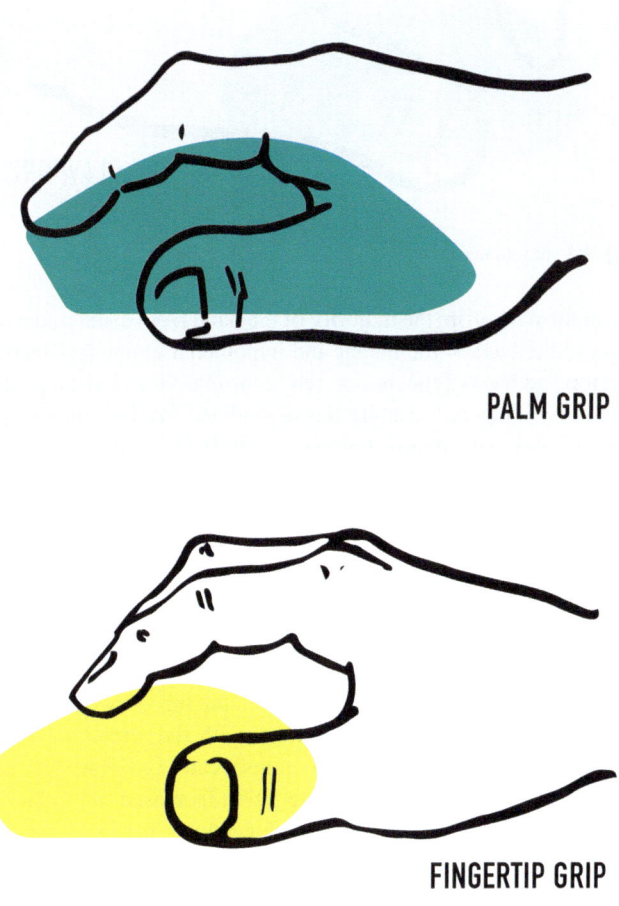

PALM GRIP

FINGERTIP GRIP

Fig. 5.2 The most common mouse grip styles utilized while gaming

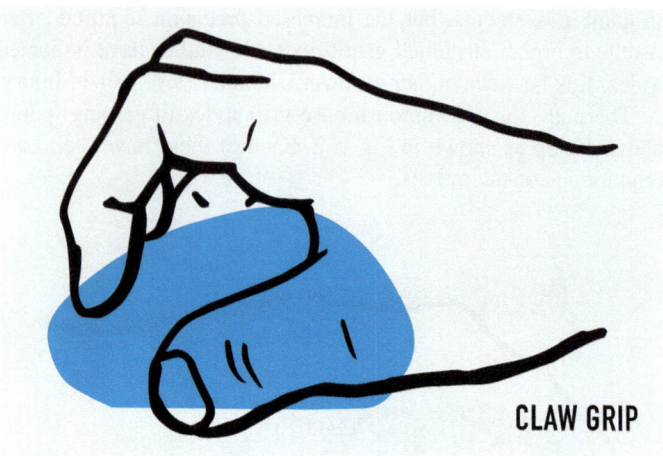

CLAW GRIP

Fig. 5.2 (continued)

In the palm grip, the majority of the hand from distal transverse arch to the base of the thenar and hypothenar eminences rests on the top and back of the mouse, while the middle and distal phalanges of two fingers – usually the second and third digits – rest on the left and right mouse buttons, respectively. This grip is most comfortable on a longer mouse with a moderate arch height, which usually correlates with a heavier weight of the mouse. It requires the least sustained contraction of wrist stabilizers but does not lend itself easily to picking up and moving the mouse.

The claw grip works best on a shorter mouse with a more aggressive arch height. In this grip, the base of the palm rests on the back edge of the mouse, the distal palm and proximal and middle phalanges are unsupported, and the tips of two fingers rest on the left and right mouse buttons, with the remaining fingers stabilizing the outer edges of the mouse, causing a more "clawed" hand shape. This grip is associated with increased muscular load over time relative to a palm grip but allows for increased ease picking up and moving the mouse when not in contact with a mousepad.

The tip grip provides the least passive support to the hand. In this grip, the palm is entirely elevated and only the tips of two fingers rest on the left and right mouse buttons, while the remaining fingers stabilize the outer edges of the mouse. This grip is associated with the greatest muscular load over time but also allows for a significant degree of precision and speed. Players using this grip should look for light, short, low-arched mice.

Regardless of grip type, wrist flexion/extension and wrist ulnar/radial deviation should rest in an approximately neutral position. Mild wrist extension, up to 15 °, does not pose any additional pain or musculoskeletal injury risk; similarly, mild wrist ulnar deviation of up to 5° may be a more comfortable position for some players. Increased ulnar deviation may increase risk of injury [5].

5.3.3 Keyboard

Two planes of motion of the wrist are relevant with regard to keyboard position. As with mouse position, attention must be paid to wrist flexion/extension, occurring in the frontal plane about a sagittal axis, and wrist ulnar/radial deviation, occurring in the coronal plane about a transverse axis. Both keyboard and mouse should allow for approximately neutral positioning of the wrist, with 0–15 ° of extension and 0–5 ° of ulnar deviation.

Mechanical keyboards are the most common keyboard type used in gaming. A mechanical keyboard is made with spring-activated key switches. Different switches have different characteristics concerning their actuation, tactile, and reset points. A keyboard's actuation point is the point at which the contact mechanism registers a key press. Tactile point is the point during the keypress at which the key provides tactile feedback to your finger that the key has been actuated, usually at the point of maximum depression. Reset points is the point at which the mechanism ceases to register the key press.

Actuation force has been shown to be correlated with musculoskeletal symptoms among office-working populations, although less research has been conducted in gaming populations. Research indicates that an actuation force of <47 cN is correlated with decreased fingertip force and electromyography activity relative to a higher actuation force [6]. Additionally, computer workers reporting higher levels of musculoskeletal symptoms in the neck and back as well as in the hands demonstrated higher key strike forces than those with lower levels of symptoms [7, 8].

While research suggests that a split keyboard design may improve neutral wrist positioning, the data is unclear whether this occurs to a statistically significant effect [9, 10]. The majority of PC gamers use standard rather than split keyboards, and at this time research does not support encouraging a transition away from standard gaming keyboards.

5.3.4 Console Controller

There are a multitude of controller categories available to console games, the most common being a gamepad controller, often called a dual analog stick controller, or simply a "controller." More specialized gaming controllers are used for different gaming categories, such as fighting games and racing games.

5.3.4.1 Gamepad Controller

As with a mouse, optimal pad size and grip type will vary depending on hand shape and playstyle. However, there is less available variation in console controller size. Most gaming consoles are designed to work best with one company-branded controller; third-party controllers may cause a greater degree of lag, or delay between button input and in-game movement. For this reason, adjusting grip type is the more common adaptation.

Some pads can be modified to address spring resistance or ease of analog stick, also known as a c-stick, movement. However, regulations vary by esport as to how much modification is legal for gameplay.

A palmar grip on a controller would position the base of the sides against the thenar eminence, the palm along the first metatarsal in contact with either side of the controller, and the index fingers curved around to rest on the left and right bumpers or triggers (per player preference). The left thumb rests on the left control stick and the right thumb rests on either the right control stick or one of the four right buttons (A, B, X, and Y/triangle, circle, X, and square). This grip is similar to the one used to text on a phone in landscape orientation.

The most common claw grip maintains the same left-handed position on the controller, but alters the right hand shape, as shown in Fig. 5.3. The base of the side is tucked against the medial aspect of the thenar eminence, the right thumb rests on the right control stick, the medial side of the distal phalanx of right second digit rests on the far-right button (B or circle), and the right third digit rests on the right bumper or trigger. Another variation of a claw grip also adjusts the left hand position, with the left thumb on the D-pad, the medial side of the left second digit on the left control stick, and the left third digit on the left bumper or trigger.

Clinical Pearl
Depending on the game title, the right thumb may spend a majority of the time on the analog stick for movement or vision, or on the buttons for actions.

As with the claw grip on the mouse, claw grip on the pad or controller sacrifices comfort for precision and speed. Depending on the game played, character selection in the individual game, and personal playstyle that degree of precision may be necessary for optimal play. Little research has been done on the impact of these positions on musculoskeletal stress. We rely on biomechanical principles to consider the potential risk for pain and strain in this instance.

Character Selection and Hand Grip
In the classic fighting game Super Smash Bros. Melee, characters like Zelda or Peach are considered "floaties," or characters with low falling speed. The playstyle that best makes use of this trait places more emphasis on using aerial attacks and a larger degree of spacing between characters and less emphasis on multi-hit combinations which require more actions per minute (APM). Conversely, characters like

Fox or Falco rely heavily on quick combinations and horizontal mobility on the stage using a technique called "shining." This playstyle requires greater APM.

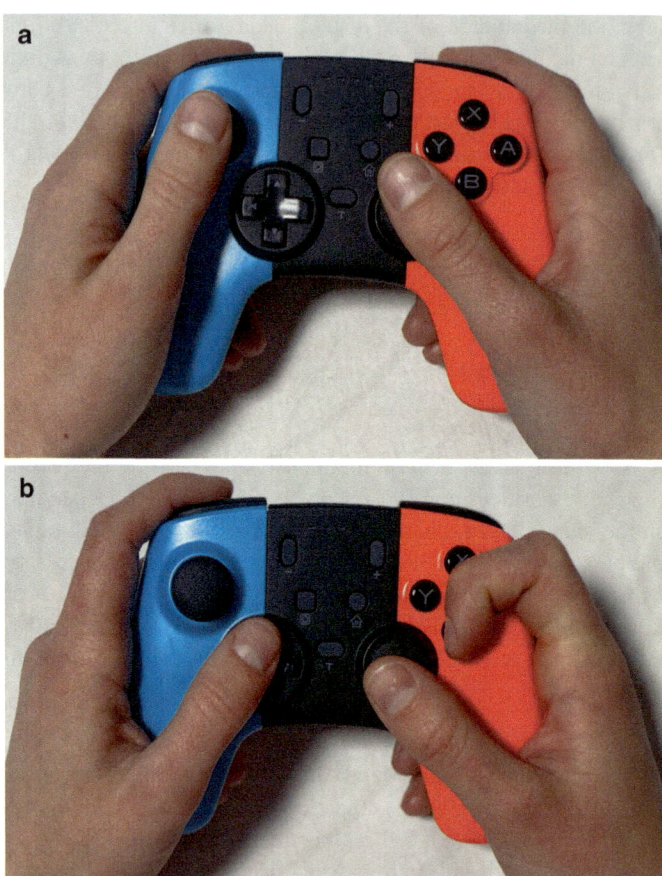

Fig. 5.3 A traditional controller grip versus the alternative "claw" grip. (**a**) In a traditional grip, both thumbs rest on the dual analog sticks, with the thumbs leaving their resting positions to reach either the D-pad or action buttons. (**b**) The claw is an alternative grip used to reach the buttons on the front side of the control, while keeping the right thumb on the analog stick

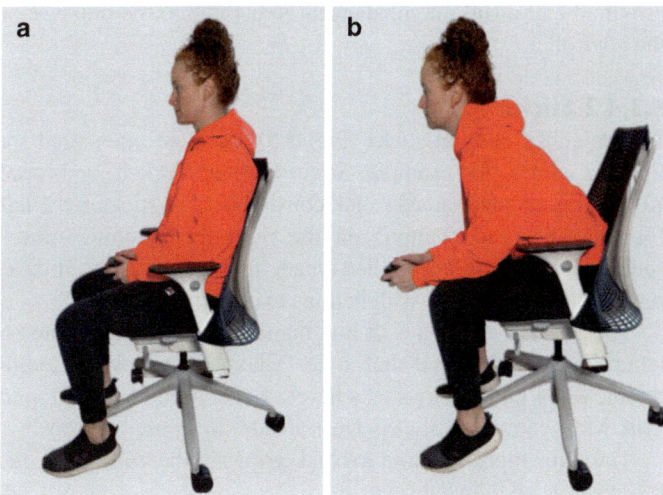

Fig. 5.4 (**a**) Optimal controller player posture with feet planted firmly on the ground, the back supported, and the controller supported by resting the forearms on the player's lap. (**b**) The common forward-leaning posture with accentuated lumbar flexion and cervical extension

The forearms are positioned in neutral supination/pronation and mild wrist extension in both positions, minimizing mechanical load for wrist extensors. If the forearms are supported on armrests or in a player's lap, forearm pronators and supinators are similarly relaxed. However, many players utilize a forward-leaning posture, as shown in Fig. 5.4, with the forearms supporting the weight of the upper body in addition to providing a stable base for mobile digits. This significantly increases forearm, upper arm, neck, and back strain over time. A better posture is one in which the player leans back, using their backrest, with forearms supported and not weight-bearing.

With the claw grip, there is a significant increase in the strain of both extrinsic and intrinsic hand muscles due to repeated flexion, extension, abduction, and adduction of the second digit. There is also strain across the collateral ligaments of both the proximal and distal interphalangeal joints due to the pressure of the controller.

5.3.4.2 Sticks

Arcade sticks or fight sticks (Fig. 5.5) are most often used for fighting games, for example, Street Fighter, Tekken, or Mortal Kombat. A standard arcade stick consists of a joystick on the left for movement and buttons on the right for inputting moves (punches, kicks, etc.). Modified arcade sticks, such as the Hitbox, replace the left joystick with buttons to control movement.

There are several ways of holding the joystick, depending on hand size, playstyle, and stick style. "Classic" joysticks are cylindrical, while ball-top joysticks have a large, round ball on top to grip. Most commercially available arcade sticks use ball-tops.

The three most common joystick grips are the wine glass, the broomstick, and the hybrid grip.

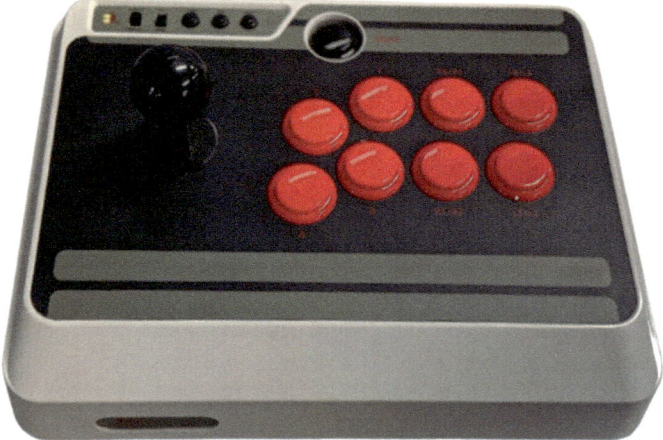

Fig. 5.5 Arcade stick. The joystick on the left traditionally controls movement, with buttons on the right for specific moves. In fighting games, specific button combinations may result in a different, more complex action than the individual buttons themselves

As with palmar and claw grips, the wine glass grip is usually more comfortable while the broomstick grip is less comfortable, but more precisely controlled. Neither grip presents a significantly elevated risk of injury or pain over the other, and player preference should guide decisions.

5.3.5 Phone and Tablet

While most research on phone and tablet ergonomics has not been specifically focused on mobile gaming ergonomics, this existing body of knowledge can inform reasonable guidelines. It is important to consider that what may be optimal ergonomically may not be optimal for player performance or precision, and that adjustments should be made on an individualized basis to meet players' competitive and ergonomic needs.

Several studies have shown the impact of phone use in sitting and in standing on neck flexion angle [11–13]. Current research suggests increased neck flexion occurs during sitting postures relative to standing postures, and that neck flexion is greatest during interactive tasks like texting. Longer durations of use are associated with greater levels of pain. Accessories such as stands and cases improve comfort and decrease excessive neck flexion postures.

Based on these data, a standing posture seems preferable for improved neck position and strain. However, without accessories, standing postures place increased loads on the hands, shoulders, and forearms to maintain the phone in a comfortable position that allows precise finger control. Additional studies indicate that forearm support is correlated with decreased musculoskeletal symptoms [14].

Different phone and tablet sizes also impact ergonomics. Larger phones or tablets requiring greater thumb reach to touch or swipe result in increased wrist extensor and flexor muscle activity, while swipe/tap locations closer to the palm where the device is stabilized allow for a more neutral thumb and wrist position and require less forearm muscle activity [15–18].

As discussed previously, continued change and adjustment is likely to be the best "posture" for mobile gaming ergonomics. Postures should include forearm support that keeps the device at a level that decreases neck flexion angle; back support that allows for a variety of forward-leaning, upright, and backward-leaning postures; and a device appropriately sized to the player, allowing for the use of either both thumbs or multiple fingers during gameplay, depending on the game.

References

1. Slater D, Korakakis V, O'Sullivan P, Nolan D, O'Sullivan K. "Sit up straight": time to re-evaluate. J Orthop Sports Phys Ther. 2019;49(8):562–4. https://doi.org/10.2519/jospt.2019.0610.
2. Sommerich CM, Joines SMB, Psihogios JP. Effects of computer monitor viewing angle and related factors on strain, performance, and preference outcomes. Hum Factors. 2001;43(1):39–55. https://doi.org/10.1518/001872001775992480.
3. Sheedy JE, Gowrisankaran S, Hayes JR. Blink rate decreases with eyelid squint. Optom Vis Sci. 2005;82(10):905–11. https://doi.org/10.1097/01.opx.0000181234.63194.a7.
4. Loh PY, Muraki S. Effect of wrist angle on median nerve appearance at the proximal carpal tunnel. PLoS One. 2015;10(2):e0117930. https://doi.org/10.1371/journal.pone.0117930.
5. Abe K, Terada N, Nakamura T. Cine MRI of the triangular fibrocartilage complex during radial–ulnar deviation. J Wrist Surg. 2018;07(04):274–80. https://doi.org/10.1055/s-0038-1668542.
6. Levanon Y, Gefen A, Lerman Y, Portnoy S, Ratzon NZ. Key strike forces and their relation to high level of musculoskeletal symptoms. Saf Health Work. 2016;7(4):347–53. https://doi.org/10.1016/j.shaw.2016.04.008.
7. Asundi K, Odell D. Effects of keyboard keyswitch design: a review of the current literature. Work. 2011;39(2):151–9. https://doi.org/10.3233/wor-2011-1161.
8. Gerard MJ, Armstrong TJ, Foulke JA, Martin BJ. Effects of key stiffness on force and the development of fatigue while typing. Am Ind Hyg Assoc J. 1996;57(9):849–54. https://doi.org/10.1080/15428119691014549.
9. Baker NA, Moehling KK, Park SY. The effect of an alternative keyboard on musculoskeletal discomfort: a randomized cross-over trial. Work. 2015;50(4):677–86. https://doi.org/10.3233/wor-131797.

10. Smith MJ, Karsh BT, Conway FT, Cohen WJ, James CA, Morgan JJ, et al. Effects of a split keyboard design and wrist rest on performance, posture, and comfort. Hum Factors. 1998;40(2):324–36. https://doi.org/10.1518/001872098779480451.

11. Douglas EC, Gallagher KM. The influence of a semi-reclined seated posture on head and neck kinematics and muscle activity while reading a tablet computer. Appl Ergon. 2015;60:342–7. https://doi.org/10.1016/j.apergo.2016.12.013.

12. Guan X, Fan G, Chen Z, Zeng Y, Zhang H, Hu A, et al. Gender difference in mobile phone use and the impact of digital device exposure on neck posture. Ergonomics. 2016;59(11):1453–61. https://doi.org/10.1080/00140139.2016.1147614.

13. Lee S, Kang H, Shin G. Head flexion angle while using a smartphone. Ergonomics. 2014;58(2):220–6. https://doi.org/10.1080/00140139.2014.967311.

14. Young JG, Trudeau MB, Odell D, Marinelli K, Dennerlein JT. Wrist and shoulder posture and muscle activity during touch-screen tablet use: effects of usage configuration, tablet type, and interacting hand. Work. 2013;45(1):59–71. https://doi.org/10.3233/wor-131604.

15. Coppola SM, Lin MYC, Schilkowsky J, Arezes PM, Dennerlein JT. Tablet form factors and swipe gesture designs affect thumb biomechanics and performance during two-handed use. Appl Ergon. 2018;69:40–6. https://doi.org/10.1016/j.apergo.2017.12.015.

16. Gustafsson E, Coenen P, Campbell A, Straker L. Texting with touch-screen and keypad phones – a comparison of thumb kinematics, upper limb muscle activity, exertion, discomfort, and performance. Appl Ergon. 2018;70:232–9. https://doi.org/10.1016/j.apergo.2018.03.003.

17. Gustafsson E. Ergonomic recommendations when texting on mobile phones. Work. 2012;41:5705–6. https://doi.org/10.3233/wor-2012-0925-5705.

18. Xiong J, Muraki S. An ergonomics study of thumb movements on smartphone touch screen. Ergonomics. 2014;57(6):943–55. https://doi.org/10.1080/00140139.2014.904007.

Nutrition for the Video Gamer

6

Lauren Trocchio

6.1 Introduction

Nutrition is well recognized as an important component of optimal sport performance, as well as promoting long-term general health for an athlete. In the last decade, esports has grown in popularity and expanded into play at the collegiate and professional levels. Given these developments, nutrition plays a performance role for the individual esports player, and ultimately, the team. Additionally, nutrition supports short- and long-term health in the setting of a nontraditional sport. Despite this, research on nutrition for esports remains almost nonexistent. Here we will consider current nutrition practices within the esports community and discuss how established guidelines on nutrition for health and performance may be applied to this population.

6.2 Basic Esports Physiology and the Role of Nutrition

Knowledge of the physical and mental demands of esports players, along with injury management, is in its infancy. However, there appear to be distinctions in the performance requirements between

L. Trocchio (✉)
Nutrition Unlocked, LLC, Arlington, VA, USA

© The Author(s), under exclusive license to Springer Nature Switzerland AG 2021
L. Migliore et al. (eds.), *Handbook of Esports Medicine*,
https://doi.org/10.1007/978-3-030-73610-1_6

most traditional sports and esports. Specifically, esports requires less physicality and greater mental performance. These distinctions may help determine appropriate nutritional management.

6.2.1 Physicality

During esports practice and competition, physicality is minimal. Energy demands, long-term metabolic and health concerns, and injury risks are likely more similar to a desk worker [1, 2]. Quantitative data on activity levels of esports athletes, whether during play or activity/exercise outside of play, is limited. One study assessed the energy expenditure of 100 young adults playing video games using indirect calorimetry. Games using traditional controllers showed a 23% increase in energy expenditure above rest versus an active dance game exhibiting a 298% increase above rest [3]. While this population was not elite esport athletes, it suggests esports play does not contribute to significant energy expenditure.

Considering alternate activity, a survey of elite or professional esports athletes found that 88.7% participated in some form of physical exercise, and 55% believed exercise could impact their esports performance. Of those participating in exercise, 47% did so for overall health reasons. The average training for surveyed athletes was just over 5 h per day, including 1 h of physical exercise [4]. This study, while small and singular, suggests the majority of esports athletes are participating in physical exercise; however, they are also spending several hours per day in a physically inactive state while training for their sport. Furthermore, other studies have reported daily gaming time up to 12 h [5].

As inactivity is linked to negative health impacts, such as insulin resistance and excess weight gain leading to overweight or obesity, nutrition may play a role in mitigating short-and long-term health risks [6]. Weight management is dependent upon achieving caloric balance between energy intake and energy expenditure, while the type or quality of calories may impact other health parameters and/or body composition. General nutrition recommendations for esports players are summarized in Table 6.1.

Table 6.1 General nutrition recommendations for esports player health (Adapted from the U.S. Dietary Guidelines 2015–2020 [7])

Choose a balanced, sustainable eating pattern that supports healthy body weight and adequate nutrition intake, which may include:
A variety of vegetables and fruits
Grains, at least half of which are whole
Reduced-fat dairy
A variety of lean animal proteins and/or plant-based protein sources, such as legumes, nuts, seeds, and soy products
Oils
Prioritize nutrient-dense foods.
Minimize added sugars and saturated fats.
When of age, only consume alcohol in moderation – up to one drink per day in women and two drinks per day in men.
Athletes eliminating food groups based on medical conditions or preference should work with a registered dietitian to ensure nutritional needs are met.

6.2.2 Cognition

While all sport participation requires some analytic component, cognitive capabilities is a critical factor in esports success. Optimal performance requires coordination, quick reaction time, manual dexterity, visual acuity, and mental focus, along with the ability to strategize and function within a team [8]. High-level esports athletes have been observed to make ten action moves per second or 500–600 moves per minute [2]. With play occurring from 3 to 10 h per day, fatigue can occur at a central, neurological level involving brain mechanisms [9, 10]. Nutrition has the potential to support cognitive function and optimal energy levels during play, but specific mechanisms have yet to be elucidated. Causative studies are challenging to conduct due to the complexity of the brain and assessing human behavior, and most research to date has been conducted in the aging population. Nevertheless, current data suggests nutrition can play a role, either positive or negative, in cognition.

Nutrients consumed from foods are the building block of neuronal pathways in the brain. Neurotransmitters responsible for chemical communications can impact cognitive performance when deficient. Choline and the amino acids tryptophan, tyrosine, phenylalanine, arginine, and threonine are all precursors for neurotransmitters and have been investigated in relationship to cognitive performance [11].

Specific macronutrient combinations to enhance cognition have not been identified; however, glucose (or glycogen) is the primary fuel source for the brain with a daily intake of up to 130 grams. Use of glucose in the brain appears to increase proportionately with task difficulty [12]. Given the mental performance aspect of esports play, glucose likely plays an important role. Despite this, research specific to this population and precise intake recommendations are both lacking. Several studies on the use of carbohydrate mouth-rinse in endurance athletes participating in activity of 45–60 min in duration have suggested an ergogenic effect activated in reward centers of the brain triggered by carbohydrate in the oral cavity [10]. While esports athletes are not engaged in endurance exercise during play, it highlights the complexity of carbohydrate's potential role in cognitive function and performance. However, a study of chess players, a sport potentially similar in mental tasking, assessing respiratory ratio during play, found it decreased over the duration (from 0.89 to 0.75), reflecting a decrease in carbohydrate substrate usage [13]. Clearly, the precise recommended dietary composition for esports players remains unknown. However, meal consumption in general may have performance benefits. Research in school-aged children has shown a positive association between breakfast intake and the ability to correctly complete complex mental functions [14].

Despite the potential cognitive benefit of carbohydrates, diets with excess added sugar are associated with increased oxidative stress and reduced synaptic plasticity [15]. Additionally, there is a small but inconclusive amount of evidence indicating low glycemic index carbohydrates (a method of measuring carbohydrate quality) are favorable towards cognitive function, but primarily in adults. Excess saturated fat and excess overall calorie intake are also associated with elevated oxidative stress and postprandial drowsiness, respectively [11]. Contrarily, unsaturated fats, specifically omega-3 docosahexaenoic acid (DHA) and eicosapen-

Table 6.2 Potential nutrition strategies for optimizing cognitive function in esports athletes

Limit foods high in saturated fat. Encourage unsaturated fats with a preference for those high in omega-3 fatty acids.
Optimize carbohydrate intake, with the goal of preventing both inadequate and excess intake.
Consider quality of the carbohydrate. Focus on sources that are higher in fiber and lower in added sugar.
Appropriately time meal and snack intakes throughout the day and during play.
Consume a variety of fruits and vegetables.
Promote euhydration with adequate fluid intake.

taenoic acid (EPA), provide building material to the brain and support synaptic signaling [14].

Finally, hydration status and the plant chemicals polyphenols have been implicated in preventing central fatigue and promoting brain health, respectively. Moderate dehydration has been associated with reduced planning and visuospatial processing, along with increased neuronal activity to perform the same cognitive functions as in a euhydrated state [14]. Polyphenols, of which the three main types are flavonoids, phenolic acids, and stilbenes, are plant micronutrients exerting antioxidant and neuroprotective effects in the brain [10]. They are found abundantly in fruits and vegetables with skin or flesh color being a common indicator of polyphenol type.

Nutrition strategies for optimizing cognition in esports athletes can be found in Table 6.2. Supplementation will be discussed in a later section.

6.3 General Nutrition

6.3.1 Macronutrients

Macronutrients are calorie-providing nutrients in the diet and consist of carbohydrate, protein, and fat. While water is considered a macronutrient due to the volume in which humans need it, it does not provide calories. Each macronutrient has purposes in health and sports performance, and individuals need them in varying amounts based on activity type, volume, and intensity; training periodization; body composition goals; and disease states [16]. While the energy expenditure and macronutrient need for esports athletes have not been systematically researched or established, the underlying purpose of macronutrients (Table 6.3) may provide insight into suggested intake amounts, sources, and timing.

6.3.2   Micronutrients

Micronutrients are nutrients needed in smaller daily amounts. They include vitamins and minerals consumed in the diet, or potentially via supplementation. At this time, it is unknown if esports athletes are at increased risk of deficiency in any particular micronutrient, and the specific role and recommended intake amount of each vitamin and mineral is beyond the scope of this chapter. It is likely that, given the indoor nature of the sport, vitamin D deficiency may occur [16]. Beyond that, deficiency risk and occurrence may depend upon individual diets and medical histories. Consuming a variety of foods may support adequate micronutrient intake. Therefore, individuals eliminating food groups due to medical reasons or preference should work with a physician and dietitian to ensure micronutrient levels are assessed and needs remain met.

6.4   Daily Fueling

Athletes may approach their fueling tactics via addressing daily fueling habits (i.e., meals and snacks) and fueling specifically around training (i.e., before, during, and after). Energy and macronutrient needs will vary by individual, and specific recommendations may be best achieved by working with a registered dietitian specializing in sports performance. For general education on intake recommendations, a performance plate is a practical, visual tool that can be used with athletes [17]. By varying the proportionate amount of certain foods on the plate, an athlete can adjust overall energy intake and macronutrient

Table 6.3 Macronutrient purposes and sources adapted from [9, 16, 27]

	Purpose	Sources	Notes
Protein	Building block of tissue, enzymes, and hormones Substrates for muscle protein synthesis	Chicken, turkey Beef, pork Fish, shellfish Dairy, eggs Soy products Legumes Nuts/seeds	Lean animal proteins are lower in saturated fat. Protein is a satiating nutrient and helps manage hunger. Protein combined with carbohydrate slows digestion and reduces spikes in blood sugar.
Carbohydrate	Anaerobic and aerobic energy source Primary fuel for high-intensity activity lasting 15 s to 2 to 3 min Rate-limiting substrate in prolonged activity Primary fuel for the brain and central nervous system Blood sugar maintenance	Bread Pasta Oatmeal, cold cereals Rice, barley, quinoa Starchy vegetables (potatoes, corn, peas, winter squash) Fruit, fruit juice Crackers, pretzels, popcorn Dairy (milk, yogurt) Legumes (beans, lentils) Sweets	Carbohydrate-containing foods are also important sources of fiber, vitamins, and minerals. Whole grain versions of foods (whole wheat bread, pasta, etc.) may provide greater nutritional value, slow digestion, and reduce spikes in blood sugar.
Fat	Aerobic energy source Primary fuel for low to moderate intensity activity Component of cellular membranes Cushions organs	Oils Avocado Nuts, seeds Fatty fish (salmon, mackerel, anchovies) Butter Sweets	Most foods with fat contain a combination of types (unsaturated, saturated). Unsaturated fats may be less inflammatory than saturated.

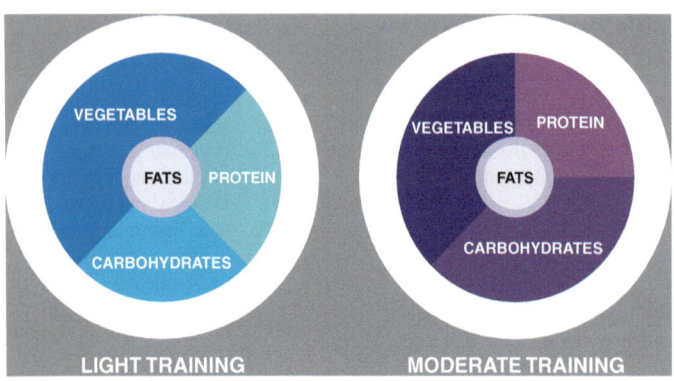

Fig. 6.1 Performance plates with ideal macronutrient balances for light training days versus moderate training days. When effort and output increase, athletes must increase carbohydrate intake appropriately, and adjust protein and vegetable intake accordingly

content to support varying levels of training (Fig. 6.1). Additionally, given the potential variability in physical activity of individual esports athletes, the plate models may facilitate educating either an individual or group, regardless of differences in activity.

When making nutrition recommendations, it is important to remember that individuals do not consume macronutrients, but rather foods. These foods consist of varying forms of individual macronutrients (i.e., carbohydrate as glucose versus fiber) with varying impacts in the body, along with containing additional nutrients such as vitamins and minerals and antioxidants. For example, whole wheat bread provides not only carbohydrate but also greater fiber and protein content than white bread. Therefore, certain foods may be preferred sources of macronutrients for both health and performance reasons, and examples are shown in Table 6.4. It is suggested individuals predominantly consume these more nutrient-dense foods; however, there remains room in a balanced diet for less nutritious but perhaps favorite or preferred foods.

The practical application of the plate method requires consideration of many individual and environmental factors. A player's

Table 6.4 Example meal combinations

Eggs + cheese + spinach + English muffin
Oatmeal + milk + peanut butter + banana
Smoothie: Protein powder + banana + blueberries + low-fat milk + flax seeds
Greek yogurt + berries + granola + almonds
Peanut butter and jelly sandwich + apple + low-fat milk
Bowl dish: Beans + cheese + brown rice + fajita vegetables (pepper, onion, mushroom) + guacamole
Whole wheat pasta + chicken sausage + tomatoes, onions, zucchini + olive oil
Wrap: Rotisserie chicken + romaine salad + whole wheat wrap + hummus
Sandwich: Roast beef + lettuce, tomato + mayo + whole wheat bread + carrot sticks
Vegetarian chili + whole grain crackers
Hamburger: Lean ground beef + lettuce, tomato + whole wheat bun + asparagus
Whole wheat toast + avocado + eggs + spinach
Bowl dish: Tofu + brown rice + stir-fry vegetables (celery, bok choy, broccoli) + sesame oil

living situation, kitchen capabilities, and culinary skills will affect the breadth of meals they are able to produce. For team houses, food choices may be largely influenced by other players, rather than individual player preference. Other concerns, such as budget, time constraints, and proximity to groceries stores, should also be evaluated. While some choices might be available at home on training days, options may be limited at the site of competition. Providers working with esports athletes regarding meal planning should consider these factors in order to develop effective recommendations (Table 6.5).

6.5   Fueling Timing

The recommended type of foods and amount consumed must be coupled with the timing of intake in order to promote optimum impact to performance [16]. Fueling before, during, and after a

Table 6.5 Fueling timing recommendations (Adapted from Burke and Deakin 27; Thomas et al. [16])

	Goals	Specific timing and strategy	Examples
Before	Prevent hypo- or hyperglycemia Establish euhydration Prevent excessive need to urinate during play Prevent excessive hunger during play Mitigate gastrointestinal distress which may occur due to performance anxiety Include foods important to the athlete's pre-event routine	**Meals** 1–4 h before play Avoid excessively large meals **Snacks** 30–60 min before play Combination of protein, carbohydrate, fat Complex carbohydrates to mitigate blood sugar spikes **Fluids** Consume fluids in 4 h leading up to play Sipping fluids and consuming with electrolytes and macronutrients to enhance retention	**Meals** See Table 5 **Snacks** Peanut butter and jelly sandwich Apple + peanut butter Turkey + English muffin Oatmeal + milk Protein + carbohydrate bar Protein + carbohydrate drink

During	Prevent hypo- or hyperglycemia during play	**Meals**	**Meals**
		Every 3–4 h during play	See Table 5
	Maintain euhydration	Avoid excessively large meals	**Snacks**
	Prevent excessive need to urinate during play	Individualize timing and portions to the athlete preference	Protein + carbohydrate drink
			Protein + carbohydrate bar
	Prevent fatigue related to CNS mechanisms	**Snacks**	Peanut butter and jelly sandwich
		Intersperse between meals as needed	Nut butter packets
	Prevent excessive hunger during play	Combination of protein, carbohydrate, fat	
	Include foods easy to consume during play	Liquid or "all-in-one" snack ideas may be easiest to consume	
		Nonperishable items may be preferred if temperature-controlled storage is unavailable	
		Fluids	
		Consume fluids periodically during play	
		Sipping fluids and consuming with electrolytes and macronutrients may enhance retention	
		Individual fluid plans may be based on urine color and developed through practice	

(continued)

Table 6.5 (continued)

	Goals	Specific timing and strategy	Examples
After	Consume meals and snacks to support total daily energy/macronutrient needs Rehydration	**Meals** Timing can align with next appropriate meal time, supporting goal of every 3–4 h Avoid meals within 1–2 h of bedtime to reduce sleep disruption **Snacks** Include a snack as needed; may be appropriate if great than 2 h before meal time Larger snack may replace meal if too close to bedtime Combination of protein, carbohydrate, fat	**Meals** See Table 5 **Snacks** Cereal + milk Chocolate milk + fruit Yogurt + granola + fruit Apple + cheese stick + almonds Hardboiled eggs + Banana 6″ cheese quesadilla English muffin + almond butter Trail mix Protein + carbohydrate drink Protein + carbohydrate bar

Table 6.6 Considerations for esports fueling timing

Pre-Fueling

What time does training or competition commence? When will the athlete wake and be ready to eat?

Does the athlete have a sensitive gastrointestinal tract, or does anxiety contribute to gastrointestinal issues? What foods are tolerated before competition?

Is training or competition near the home where commonly consumed foods are available? If traveling, how will the athlete acquire food – at the competition site, or on his/her own?

During Fueling

How often will the athlete be able to stop play in order to eat or drink?

Is the athlete concerned with the frequency of needing to use the restroom during play?

Is the food easy to handle and avoids hand residue?

What foods will be accessible? Does the athlete need to pack snacks for training or competition?

Post-Fueling

What did the athlete consume before and during training or competition?

What foods are accessible to the athlete?

workout or competition in traditional sports has specific purposes. The ideal fueling timing specifically around esports play and competition remains unexplored in research; however, the application of traditional sport fueling and general health may guide recommendations (Table 6.6). The goals and content as noted are limited to what may apply in the esports setting. Should esports athletes partake in additional exercise, in particular at volumes greater than 1 h per day or at higher intensity, further fueling recommendations may apply.

Similar to meal planning, the practical application of fueling timing requires consideration of many individual and environmental factors, in particular those that may be specific to the esports environment. Providers working with esports athletes regarding meal planning should consider these factors in order to develop effective recommendations (Table 6.6).

6.6 Supplements

Supplement use is widespread across sports and the general population. In traditional sport settings, athletes describe using supplements for general health purposes, the management of known micronutrient deficiencies, and the enhancement of performance through benefits like physique alteration, recovery support, and the management of pain and injuries [18]. There is also specific interest in supplementation for enhanced cognitive function, which is of particular interest in the esports population [10]. Minimal data on effectiveness of supplementation for esports performance or esports athlete supplementation usage exists. Commercial products and marketing towards the esports community, along with anecdotal observation at competitions, suggests enhanced cognitive performance through the use of supplements is of interest. However, research on supplementation in traditional sport settings may be hard to apply to esports as confounders like exercise and environmental conditions such as temperature and altitude may alter the impact to the brain.

Supplements purported to enhance cognitive performance are likely of most interest to esport athletes. Here we will consider them as categories of stimulants or nootropics, along with those supporting vision health.

6.6.1 Stimulants

The primary supplement within this category is caffeine, which has been well established as having benefits for athletic performance, including improved alertness and vigilance [18, 19]. Guarana, which contains caffeine, should be considered as well. Despite heavy marketing of energy drinks to esports athletes, data specific to the esports population is limited. A lone reported randomized control trial in elite esports players suggests the use of a commercially available energy drink provides no benefit to performance [16]. Additionally, ideal intake amounts of caffeine are unknown in a nontraditional sport setting. Metabolization of caffeine is individual, and excess intake is associated with negative side effects, such as nausea, irritability, sleep disruption, and diuresis [18, 19]. Esports athletes considering caffeine use for performance benefits should work with a dietitian to determine the appropriate amount and timing, along with avoidance of negative side effects.

6.6.2 Nootropics

Nootropics are a wide variety of substances that may be used as cognitive enhancers. These substances may be prescription drugs or supplements, the latter of which are commonly herbal or plant ingredients. Some examples are acetyl L-carnitine, ginkgo, ginseng, St. John's wort, ashwagandha, ginseng, and L-theanine. To date, the majority of research on such substances has been conducted in the aging population [10]. There is currently not enough evidence to support the broad use of any herbal or plant-based nootropic supplement, and well-controlled, quality data specifically on esports athlete performance is lacking.

Nitric oxide has gained some interest for its ability to improve cognitive performance [20]. Beetroot juice is the commonly used delivery system as it is high in inorganic nitrate, which converts to nitric oxide and improves endothelial function, oxygen delivery, and cerebral blood flow [10]. However, research has mostly been performed in athletes performing physical exercise; therefore, an accurate assessment of nitric oxide's impact to cognitive performance in esports athletes cannot be made at this time.

6.6.3 Vision Health

Given the propensity for eye fatigue and strain during prolonged esports play, there may be interest in supplementation to support vision health [1, 2]. At this time, there is a lack of research on supplementation for vision health to provide recommendations for esports athletes.

6.6.4 Supplement Safety

Effectiveness is one factor in the decision to take a supplement. The other primary factor involves assessing supplement safety. In the United States, under the Dietary Supplement Health and Education Act of 1994 (DSHEA), supplements are regulated by the Food and Drug Administration (FDA) but in a different manner than pharmaceuticals or food. The responsibility of appropriate labeling and the safety of supplements falls to the manufacturers with no requirement for third-party pre-market approval. The FDA is responsible for taking action against supplements which are found to have safety concerns or mislabeling once already on the market. This regulatory gap leads to potential risks with supplement use, such as unlisted ingredients in a product, inaccurate amounts of products listed as ingredients, or contaminants such as metals [18]. This has safety concerns, but athletes subject to drug testing must also be aware of the potential for a supplement to contain substances banned by their regulatory body.

There are multiple esports leagues with varying regulatory agencies. While most do not have a banned substance list similar to one applied to NCAA and Olympic athletes, some are beginning to introduce lists of substances prohibited for use without therapeutic exemption. The majority of prohibited substances are prescription stimulants, specifically amphetamines [21]. Given the increased awareness of performance-enhancing substances and developing policies on their use, esports athletes should be aware of the risk of supplements containing banned ingredients, in addition to overall safety concerns. Third-party testing companies have been developed in order to assess supplement ingredients, and athletes may benefit from choosing supplements that have undergone these evaluations. Two such companies are NSF International Certified for Sport® and Informed Choice© [22, 23].

6.7 Special Considerations

Population characteristics of sports may give insight into considerations one should make when working with athletes. While esports research is in its infancy, some characteristics are emerging. Exploring these on an individual athlete level may enhance the applicability of nutrition research and recommendations. Examples include:

- Sleep: Initial evidence suggests the nature of esports play and training may promote disruptions to circadian rhythm and the sleep cycle [24]. Sleep alterations may not only impact esports performance, but general health.
- Gender: Current data suggests more males than females participate in esports play, in particular at the elite level [25, 26]. Application of current and future research on nutrition for health and esports performance must consider any potential differences in outcomes based on the study population (male versus female).
- Age: Current data indicates esports athletes are a younger population, with elite players ranging from early teens to late twenties, and may vary by league [1]. Nutrition recommendations to support appropriate life span and life skills will be necessary.
- Other training: Evidence suggests elite esports athletes may participate in physical training outside of sport play [1, 4]. Such training must be considered when developing fueling recommendations.

6.8   Summary

Esports has developed into an internationally recognized, elite-level sport with unique training and competition demands. Further research is needed in this population to better understand nutrition practices and needs; however, general public health messages regarding diet and activity level may be applicable given the similarities in physicality between esports and desk workers. Nutrition to enhance cognitive performance may be the primary interest for esports athletes. Further evidence is needed to suggest specific dietary content and timing modifications along with supplementation to support optimal esports play.

References

1. DiFrancisco-Donoghue J, Balentine J, Schmidt G, Zaibel H. Managing the health of the eSport athlete: an integrated health management model. BMJ Open Sport Exerc Med. 2019;5:1–6. https://doi.org/10.1136/bmjsem-2018-000467.
2. Zwibel H, DiFrancisco-Donoghue J, DeFeo A, Yao S. An osteopathic physician's approach to the eSports athlete. J Am Osteopath Assoc. 2018;119(11):756–62. https://doi.org/10.7556/jaoa.2019.125.
3. Lyons EJ, Tate DF, Ward DS, Bowling JM, Ribisit KM, Kayararaman S. Energy expenditure and enjoyment during video game play: differences by game type. Med Sci Sports Exerc. 2011;43(10):1987–93. https://doi.org/10.1249/MSS.0b013e318216ebf3.
4. Kari T, Karhulahti VM. Do e-athletes move? A study on training and physical exercise in elite eSports. Int J Gaming Comput Mediat Simul. 2016;8(4):53–66. https://doi.org/10.4018/IJGCMS.2016100104.
5. Thomas CJ, Rothschild J, Earnest CP, Blaisdell A. The effects of energy drink consumption on cognitive and physical performance in elite League of Legends players. Sports. 2019;7(9):196–205. https://doi.org/10.3390/sports7090196.
6. Bird SR, Hawley JA. Update on the effects of physical activity on insulin sensitivity in humans. BMJ Open Sport Exerc Med. 2016;2(1):1–26. https://doi.org/10.1136/bmjsem-2016-000143.
7. U.S. Department of Health and Human Services. Physical activity guidelines for Americans. 2nd ed. Washington, DC; 2018.
8. Steinkuhler C. Esports research: critical, empirical, and historical studies of competitive videogame play. Games Cult. 2020;15(1, 3):–8. https://doi.org/10.1177/0193723518773287.
9. Burke L, Hawley JA. Swifter, higher, stronger: what's on the menu? Science. 2018;362:781–7. https://doi.org/10.1126/science.aau2093.
10. Meeusen R, Decroix L. Nutritional supplements and the brain. Int J Sport Nutr. 2018;28(2):200–11. https://doi.org/10.1123/ijsnem.2017-0314.
11. Lieberman HR. Nutrition, brain function and cognitive performance. Appetite. 2003;40:245–54. https://doi.org/10.1016/s0195-6663(03)00010-2.
12. Messier C. Glucose improvement of memory: a review. Eur J Pharmacol. 2004;490(1):33–57. https://doi.org/10.1016/j.ejphar.2004.02.043.
13. Troubat N, Fargeas-Gluck MA, Tulppo M, Dugue B. The stress of chess players as a model to study the effects of psychological stimuli on physiological responses: an example of substrate oxidation and heart rate variability in man. Eur J Appl Physiol. 2009;105:343–9. https://doi.org/10.1007/s00421-008-0908-2.
14. Meeusen R. Exercise, nutrition and the brain. Sports Med. 2014;44(Suppl 1):47–56. https://doi.org/10.1007/s40279-014-0150-5.

15. Gomez-Pinilla F. The combined effects of exercise and foods in prevention neurological and cognitive disorders. Prev Med. 2011;52:S75–80. https://doi.org/10.1016/j.ypmed.2011.01.023.
16. Thomas D, Erdman K, Burke L. Position of the academy of nutrition and dietetics, dietitians of Canada, and the American College of Sports Medicine: nutrition and athletic performance. J Acad Nutr Diet. 2016;116(3):501–28. https://doi.org/10.1016/j.jand.2015.12.006.
17. Reguant-Closa A, Harris MM, Lohman TG, Meyer NL. Validation of the athlete's plate nutrition educational tool: phase 1. Int J Sport Nutr. 2019;29:628–35. https://doi.org/10.1123/ijsnem.2018-0346.
18. Maughan R, Burke L, Dvorak J, Larson-Meyer D, Peeling P, Phillips S, et al. IOC consensus statement: dietary supplements and the high-performance athlete. Br J Sports Med. 2018;52(7):439–55. https://doi.org/10.1136/bjsports-2018-099027.
19. Goldstein E, Ziegenfuss T, Kalman D, Kreider R, Campbell B, Wilborn C, et al. International society of sports nutrition position stand: caffeine and performance. J Int Soc Sports Nutr. 2010;7(5) https://doi.org/10.1186/1550-2783-7-5.
20. Tartar J, Kalman D, Hewlings S. A prospective study evaluating the effects of a nutritional supplement intervention on cognition, mood states, and mental performance in video gamers. Nutrients. 2019;11(10):2326–22340. https://doi.org/10.3390/nu11102326.
21. ESIC eSports Prohibited List 2016. Esports Integrity Commission, United Kingdom. https://esic.gg/codes/esic-prohibited-list/. Accessed 8 Apr 2020
22. Informed Choice: Trusted by Sport. https://www.informed-choice.org/. Accessed 8 Apr 2020
23. NSF International Certified for Sport. https://www.nsfsport.com/. Accessed 8 Apr 2020
24. Bonnar D, Castine B, Kakoschke N, Sharp G. Sleep and performance in Eathletes: for the win! Sleep Health. 2019;5(6):647–50. https://doi.org/10.1016/j.sleh.2019.06.007.
25. Reitman JG, Anderson-Coto MJ, Wu M, Lee JS, Steinkuehler C. Esports research: a literature review. Games Cult. 2020;15(1):32–50. https://doi.org/10.1177/1555412019840892.
26. Ruvalcaba O, Shulze J, Kim A, Berzenski S, Otten MP. Women's experiences in eSports: gendered differences in peer and spectator feedback during competitive video game play. J Sport Soc Issues. 2018;42(4):295–311.
27. Burke L, Deakin V. Clinical sports nutrition. 4th ed. Australia: McGraw-Hill; 2010.

The Psychology of Digital Games

7

Rachel Kowert
and Christopher Ferguson

7.1 Introduction

Interest in the impact of game play on the psychological well-being of players has been evident since the development of the first recreational video game. Concerns of "electronic friendships," "murder simulators," and "addictive technology" remain just as prevalent today as they did when these concerns were first discussed in public discourse [1–4].

Over the last several decades, the study of games has grown into a multidisciplinary effort, with researchers from psychology, sociology, anthropology, communication science, and media studies (among others) pooling their efforts to better understand how this digital technology impacts the physical, social, and psychological well-being of its players.

This chapter will explore some of the primary concerns relating to the psychological impact of games. Specifically, it will

R. Kowert (✉)
TakeThis, Seattle, WA, USA
e-mail: rachel@takethis.org

C. Ferguson
Department of Psychology, Stetson University, DeLand, FL, USA
e-mail: cjfergus@stetson.edu

© The Author(s), under exclusive license to Springer Nature
Switzerland AG 2021
L. Migliore et al. (eds.), *Handbook of Esports Medicine*,
https://doi.org/10.1007/978-3-030-73610-1_7

discuss the relationships between video game content and behavior change (i.e., aggression and violence and behavioral addiction) and cognitive change (i.e., impact on mental well-being and skill development). Special attention will also be given to the newly designated Gaming Disorder (GD) as put forward by the World Health Organization in the International Classification of Diseases-11 (ICD-11) [4]. The discussions will begin with a brief overview of the rise of the video game industry and its corresponding moral panic.

7.2   The Rise of the Video Game Panic

Since the advent of the telegraph, popular media has approached new forms of technology with suspicion. Video games are no exception, as controversial debates about them have been evident since their introduction in the 1970s [5]. Online video games incited a new range of concerns, as parents and researchers alike continue to express their apprehension over the potential negative consequences of prolonged use of online games.

For numerous reasons, perhaps in part because of its rapid growth, online gaming is an activity that has become highly stereotyped. That is, it is an activity that has come to be associated in popular culture with a highly specific, caricatured, and often negative image [6–8]. This depiction has been reflected in numerous television shows, news reports, current affairs programs, and other sources of popular culture. As Williams et al. states, "game players are stereotypically male and young, pale from too much time spent indoors and socially inept. ...young male game players are far from aspirational figures" [8]. The negative characterizations of game players have been further sensationalized by news reports focusing on the potential consequences of this activity. Popular news media often highlight the problematic and addictive nature of online video games, and a variety of Internet websites, magazine articles, and news articles dispense advice for individuals with problematic playing behaviors. When a violent act is committed by a young person, video games remain one of the first scapegoats.

Media portrayals and news reports have presented a consistent and negative image of video game players since their inception – they are unpopular at best and obsessive, socially inept, and reclusive at worst [7, 9]. Beyond that, gaming itself has been presented as a dangerous activity that may lead to social withdrawal, declining physical and mental health, and even murderous rage.

However, the empirical research in this area paints a far more nuanced story. For example, despite the negative characterizations in the media, research has found online gamers to be no more or less overweight, socially isolated, or unambitious than their non-game playing counterparts [9]. Links between violent video games and violent crime is also not as straightforward, and in fact, direct links between games and violence have yet to be demonstrated despite thousands of research papers published in this area. Taking a closer look at the research, it becomes clear that the moral panic surrounding video games is exactly just that – a panic based on changing technology and what is being perceived as a shift in "morals," rather than measurable behavioral and cognitive changes. This is discussed in more detail below.

7.3   Behavioral and Cognitive Impact of Digital Games

Concerns about the impact of video games have focused around behavioral and cognitive change. The primary concerns about behavior change have revolved around the impact of violent video games on aggression and violent crime and the potential for video games to contribute to behavioral addiction. In regard to cognitive change, there has been a lot of concern regarding the impact of digital game play on psychological well-being. While this ties in with talks about video game addiction and/or gaming disorder, there have been broader concerns as to how engaging in online game play may contribute to feelings of depression, loneliness, and social anxiety.

Conversely, over the last few years, there has been a bit of a shift in the study of digital games to include analyses of the potential positive cognitive impact they may be having, in terms of the ways in which games can encourage and support skill development.

Each of these topics will be discussed in more detail in the following sections.

7.4   Aggression and Violent Crime

The concern about the impact of video games on aggressive behavior and violent crime can be traced back to the popularization of the media itself. In 1976, Death Race (Exidy) was released and met with immediate skepticism and criticism about the impact of its content on players. These concerns have not abandoned and continue to grow in conjunction with the growth in accessibility of video games and more realistic graphics. Today, in the twenty-first century, we continue to hear politicians in the United States criticize video games and video games makers for creating "death simulators."

However, the research paints quite a different story. In fact, of the hundreds of studies that have been conducted looking at violent video games and violent crime, not a single one has found a direct link [10].

The links with video game play and milder aggression (such as giving someone spicy food or bursts of annoying noise) are a little more nuanced. There are some research studies that have found small (but significant) links between violent video game play and increased aggression in laboratory studies. However, other studies have not found such effects. Further, there are substantial limitations to this work that must be considered.

First, these studies have all been conducted in highly controlled laboratory environments, making it difficult to generalize to real-world actions and tendencies. Secondly, these studies measured short-term changes in aggression with measures with little external validity, such as word completion tasks or the aptly named "hot sauce paradigm." Third, preregistered studies, those that require scholars to publish their hypotheses and analysis plans in advance to reduce questionable researcher practices, have almost all found no evidence for links between violent games and even mild aggression [10]. This suggests that issues such as publication bias and poor researcher practices were responsible for most aggression effects, not actual relationships between games and aggression.

Hot Sauce Paradigm
Developed in 1999, the hot sauce paradigm is a laboratory method for measuring aggression in which participants are asked to administer varying amounts of "extremely spicy" hot sauce to a target, knowingly causing pain [11].

Additionally, even if these results were taken at face value, one cannot generalize small changes in aggression to tendencies to commit real-world violent crimes, such as mass shootings. Particularly, demographic factors such as violence, trait aggression, and peer delinquency have all been found to be far more influential in predicting violent behavior [12].

As such, opinions on the impact of games on aggression remain divided among scholars [13]. This likely explains why the American Psychiatric Association's (APA) own media psychology division released an open letter critiquing their position linking games to aggression as unscientific [14].

7.5 Addiction

Talk of video game addiction began to dominate the discussion of video game effects following the most recent publication of the Diagnostic and Statistical Manual of Mental Disorders published by the APA, whereby Internet gaming disorder (GD) was identified as a potential psychiatric condition that required additional research. In the same year, the Substance-Related Disorders working group also called for research assessing GDs etiology and stability [15]. Concern about problematic and addicted gaming were reinvigorated in 2016, when the World Health Organization (WHO) announced they were considering including GD in their new edition of the International Classification of

Diseases (ICD-11). This, however, resulted in some criticism with the media psychology divisions of the American Psychological Association and Psychological Society of Ireland releasing a joint public statement criticising the "gaming disorder" diagnosis as unscientific and likely to do more harm than good.

While several years have passed since this initial call for research, there remain active debates about how GD should be conceptualized and assessed; some standard practices have begun to emerge from the literature [16, 17]. Specifically, GD has come to be measured via a nine-item checklist, with the report of five or more of the nine criteria occurring over the previous year, plus an endorsement of personal distress due to Internet gaming indicating addiction [15, 17]. The nine criteria are as follows:

1. Spent too much time thinking about games
2. Felt moody or anxious when unable to play
3. Increased playtime to keep excitement high
4. Felt that I should play less but could not
5. Kept playing even though it caused problems
6. Kept others from knowing how much I play
7. Played to escape uncomfortable feelings
8. Reduced or lost interest in other activities
9. Risked friends or opportunities due to games

While the wording may vary slightly across study, the assessment of GD has consistently assessed themes of salience (video game play begins to dominate the player's thoughts, emotions, and behavior), mood modification (the player experiences a change in mood because of video game play), conflict (the player begins to suffer negative interpersonal, occupational, and psychological consequences due to game play), tolerance (the player needs increasing amounts of play time to achieve the mood-modifying effects), withdrawal (when the player is unable to play, they become frustrated and irritable) and relapse (players repeatedly fail to reduce their video game use). To qualify for a diagnosis of GD, participants will need to endorse five or more of the nine criteria (administered via checklist) and endorse the criteria of "personal distress due to gaming use" [15, 17]. Some scholars have, however, criticized these symptoms as borrowing too directly from substance abuse, and potentially resulting in a high degree of false positives [18].

Prevalence rates of GD within the general population have yet to be established making it difficult to determine the severity of the problem. Among representative adolescent samples, GD has been pinpointed at 1.6% of adolescents in Europe, between 0.2% and 1.16% German adolescents, and 3% typical among studies of American adolescents [19–22]. A 2011 meta-analysis of 33 published studies and doctoral dissertations indicated an overall prevalence rate of 3.1% [20]. This variability is due to variations in participant demographics (adolescents versus adults) and sample characteristics (opportunity or representative).

Research examining the relationship between problematic and/ or addicted game playing on the well-being of players has been limited. A 2009 study from Liu and Peng found significant relationships between online game playing and a range of negative life outcomes relating to physical, personal, and academic/professional problems. It has also been hypothesized that the relationship between poorer mental health outcomes and online video game use may also be cyclical. However, a lack of longitudinal research makes it difficult to determine the exact nature of these relationships.

A smaller amount of cross-sectional research has emerged pinpointing gaming disorder to these outcomes, including depression and anxiety, as well as other poorer mental health outcomes such as lower self-esteem and low life satisfaction [19, 23–25]. A 2010 study by Mehroof and Griffiths found significant associations between trait anxiety, state anxiety, and aggression with online gaming addiction [25]. In 2016, Kim and colleagues found individuals who were classified into a risk group for Internet gaming disorder (they met 5 or more of the 9 criteria as outlined by the DSM) scored higher on measures of depression, anxiety, phobic anxiety, interpersonal sensitivity, and hostility, among others [23]. As previously mentioned, Lemmens and colleagues found loneliness to emerge as a cause and a consequence of problematic play. Low self-esteem and low social competence were also found to predict later pathological gaming, suggesting that they are motivators of problematic play rather than consequences of engagement. This work again points to the potential cyclical nature of these relationships [26]. Interestingly, a follow-up study by Kowert and colleagues did not find these same patterns among non-disordered gamers, suggesting that the relationships uncovered by Lemmens and colleagues is specifically applicable to pathological game players rather than the online game playing community as a whole.

There have only been a handful of studies exploring the psychological consequences of GD over time [18, 26, 27]. Lemmens and colleagues found loneliness to emerge as a cause and a consequence of problematic play, indicating that lonely individuals are more likely to engage problematically and, over time, problematic use of online games contributes to increased levels of loneliness. Low self-esteem and low social competence were also found to predict later pathological gaming, suggesting that they are motivators of problematic play rather than consequences of engagement [26]. Sharkow and colleagues found relationships between problematic gaming and perceptions of success and life satisfaction [27]. Weinstein and colleagues found that a GD diagnosis did not predict lower levels of social, mental, and physical health after 6-months time [30]. As it stands today, it remains unclear whether GD undermines psychological health directly or indirectly [26, 28].

Today, there remains significant backlash from the scientific community, voicing significant concerns about the content of gaming disorder (as proposed by the ICD-11) due to the low-quality research to operationally define and monitor the proposed topic (including a lack of evidence demonstrating the impact of GD on the mental well-being of players), the operational definition of gaming disorder relying too heavily upon substance use and gambling disorder criteria, and a lack of consensus on symptomology and assessment of problematic gaming [29]. Mental health professionals are also concerned that the disordered use of gaming may not be a distinct, unique disorder at all but rather a maladaptive coping strategy for managing other underlying challenges. Additional research is needed to fully understand the scope of video game addiction and whether or not it is truly an addiction in and of itself or simply a manifestation of other psychological conditions.

7.6   Impact on Psychological Well-Being

In conjunction with discussions about gaming disorder and the impact of video games on aggression, there has been an increased interest in evaluating the general impact of video game play on well-being. Most of the attention has, perhaps, been most focused on gaming disorder and related concerns. The good news is that non-pathological gaming, including using games with violent content, does not appear to be associated with problematic mental health outcomes [30].

By contrast, some studies suggest that gaming is associated with a host of mental health benefits such as reduced stress and increased opportunities for socialization [31]. These benefits may be particularly pronounced for individuals with social or developmental issues, who may struggle to socialize in real-life situations [32]. The positive effects of well-being may also be much broader, with recent work from Kowert, demonstrating how video game play can contribute to various outcomes related to life satisfaction, including a growth mindset, mindfulness, and resilience [6].

Taken together, evidence suggests that, used in balance with other required life activities such as exercise, adequate sleep and attention to school, work, and family, video games, even action games, are largely a positive part of youth development [33].

7.7   Skill Development

Research has found that video games can contribute to improvement in a variety of cognitive skills such as visuo-spatial skills, increased attention, flexible thinking, and creativity [34–37].

Video games are effective tools for learning due to the inherent play aspect and induced state of "flow," which is a state of focused concentration that is achieved when the challenge of the in-game tasks are balanced with the skills of the player [38]. It is here that learning is optimized.

It is important not to overstate the links between games in learning as the transfer of learning from one context to another (in-game to out-of game). While this phenomenon does occur, it tends to be quite narrow. For example, players who favor sports simulator titles do not gain noticeable proficiency in that traditional sport in offline contexts. However, video games do hold the ability to hone broad skills, such as creative thinking and problem solving.

7.8   Concluding Thoughts

Concerns that video games have a deleterious impact on youth appear to be unfounded. We can be quite certain that action games play no role in causing violent crime, and even their involvement in prank-level aggression appears increasingly unlikely. Some individuals may overdo gaming, although this appears more likely to be a symptom of underlying, pre-existing disorders rather than a condition caused by games themselves. Significant evidence suggests that, used in balance with other life responsibilities, games can be a positive part of youth development. As such, the current pool of evidence suggests that youth involvement in esports can be positive for most and is no more likely to cause problems than is involvement in other sports activities.

References

1. Domahidi E, Breuer J, Kowert R, Festl R, Quandt T. A longitudinal analysis of gaming- and non-gaming-related friendships and social support among social online game players. Media Psychol. 2018;21(2):288–307. https://doi.org/10.1080/15213269.2016.1257393.
2. Grossman D. Video games as 'murder simulators' variety. 2013. https://variety.com/2013/voices/opinion/grossman-2640/. Accessed 8 Apr 2020
3. Selnow GW. Playing videogames: the electronic friend. J Commun. 1984;34(2):148–56. https://doi.org/10.1111/j.1460-2466.1984.tb02166.x.
4. World Health Organization. International classification of diseases for mortality and morbidity statistics (11th Revision). 2018. https://icd.who.int/browse11/l-m/en. Accessed 8 Apr 2020
5. Williams D. A brief social history of game play: playing video games: motives, responses, and consequences. Conference: Digital Games Research Conference. 2005. https://www.researchgate.net/

publication/221217533_A_Brief_Social_History_of_Game_Play.
Accessed 2 Feb 2021

6. Kowert R. Video games and well-being: press start. Cham: Palgrave
   Mamillian; 2020.
7. Kowert R, Oldmeadow J. (A)Social reputation: exploring the relationship
   between online video game involvement and social competence. Comput
   Hum Behav. 2013;29:1872–8.
8. Williams D, Yee N, Caplan S. Who plays, how much, and why?
   Debunking the stereotypical gamer profile. J Comput-Mediat Commun.
   2008;13 https://doi.org/10.1111/j.1083-6101.2008.00428.x.
9. Kowert R, Festl R, Quand T. Unpopular, overweight, and socially inept:
   reconsidering the stereotype of online gamers. Cyberpsychol Behav Soc
   Netw. 2014;17:141–6. https://doi.org/10.1089/cyber.2013.0118.
10. Ferguson CJ. Aggressive video games research emerges from its replica-
    tion crisis (sort of). Curr Opin Psychol. 2020;36:1–6. https://doi.
    org/10.1016/j.copsyc.2020.01.002.
11. Lieberman JD, Solomon S, Greenberg J, McGregor H. A hot new way to
    measure aggression: hot sauce allocation. Agress Behav. 1999;25(5):331–
    48.   https://doi.org/10.1002/(SICI)1098-2337(1999)25:5<331::AID-
    AB2>3.0.CO;2-1.
12. DeCamp W. Impersonal agencies of communication: comparing the
    effects of video games and other risk factors on violence. Psychol Pop
    Media Cult. 2015;4(4):296–304. https://doi.org/10.1037/ppm0000037.
13. Quandt T, Van Looy J, Vogelgesang J, Elson M, Ivory JD, Consalvo M,
    Mäyrä F. Digital games research: a survey study on an emerging field and
    its prevalent debates. J Commun. 2015;65(6):975–96.
14. Society for Media Psychology and Technology. Open letter to the
    American Psychological Association regarding their policy statement on
    violent   video   games.   2020.   https://www.scribd.com/docu-
    ment/448927394/Division-46-Letter-to-the-APA-criticizing-it-s-recent-
    review-of-video-game-violence-literature. Accessed 8 Apr 2020
15. Hasin DS, O'Brien CP, Auriacombe M, Borges G, Bucholz K, Budney
    A, et al. DSM-5 criteria for substance use disorders: recommenda-
    tions and rationale. Am J Psychol. 2013; https://doi.org/10.1176/appi.
    ajp.2013.12060782.
16. Griffiths MD, Van Rooij A, Kardefelt-Winther D, Starcevic V, Király O,
    Pallesen S, et al. Working towards an international consensus on criteria
    for assessing Internet gaming disorder: a critical commentary on Petry
    et al. (2014). Addiction. 2016;111:167–75. https://doi.org/10.1111/
    add.13057.
17. Petry NM, Rehbein F, Gentile DA, Lemmens JS, Rumpf H, Mößle T,
    et al. An international consensus for assessing internet gaming disorder
    using the new DSM-5 approach. Addiction. 2014;109:1399–406.

18. Przybylski A, Weinstein N, Murayama K. Internet gaming disorder: investigating the clinical relevance of a new phenomenon. Am J Psychiatry. 2017;174:230–6.
19. Festl R, Scharkow M, Quandt T. Problematic computer game use among adolescents, younger and older adults. Addiction. 2013;108(3):59209. https://doi.org/10.1111/add.12016.
20. Ferguson CJ, Coulson M, Barnett J. A meta-analysis of pathological gaming prevalence and comorbidity with mental health, academic and social problems. J Psychiatr Res. 2011;45(12):1573–8. https://doi.org/10.1016/j.jpsychires.2011.09.005.
21. Muller KW, Beutel ME, Egloff B, Wolfing K. Investigating risk factors for internet gaming disorder: a comparison of patients with addictive gaming, pathological gamblers and healthy controls regarding the big five personality traits. Eur Addict Res. 2014;20(3):129–36. https://doi.org/10.1159/000355832.
22. Rehbein F, Kliem S, Baier D, Mößle T, Petry NM. Prevalence of Internet gaming disorder in German adolescents: a diagnostic contribution of the nin DSM-5 criteria in a state-wide representative sample. Addiction. 2015;110(5):842–51. https://doi.org/10.1111/add.12849.
23. Kim NR, Hwang S, Choi JS, Kim D, Demetrovics Z, Kiraly O, et al. Characteristics and psychiatric symptoms of internet gaming disorder among adults using self-reported DSM-5 criteria. Psychol Invest. 2016;13(1):58. https://doi.org/10.4306/pi.2016.13.1.58.
24. Stetina BU, Kothgassner OD, Lehenbauer M, Kryspin-Exner I. Beyond the fascination of online-games: probing addictive behavior and depression in the world of online-gaming. Comput Hum Behav. 2011;27(1):473–9. https://doi.org/10.1016/j.chb.2010.09.015.
25. Mehroof M, Griffiths MD. Online gaming addiction: the role of sensation seeking, self-control, neuroticism, aggression, state anxiety, and trait anxiety. Cyberpsychol Behav Soc Netw. 2010;13(3):313–6. https://doi.org/10.1089/cyber2009.0229.
26. Lemmens JS, Valkenburg PM, Peter J. The effects of pathological gaming on aggressive behavior. J Youth Adolesc. 2011;40(1):38–47. https://doi.org/10.1007/s10964-010-9558-x.
27. Scharkow M, Festl R, Quandt T. Longitudinal patterns of problematic computer game use among adolescents and adults—a 2 year panel study. Addiction. 2014;109(11):1910–7. https://doi.org/10.1111/add.12662.
28. Mellor D, Stokes M, Firth L, Hayashi Y, Cummins R. Need for belonging, relationship satisfaction, loneliness, and life satisfaction. Personal Individ Differ. 2008;45(3):213–8. https://doi.org/10.1016/j.paid.2008.03.020.
29. Aarseth E, Bean AM, Boonen H, Colder Carras M, Coulson M, Das D, et al Scholars' open debate paper on the World Health Organization ICD-11 gaming disorder proposal (2016) J Behav Addict. https://doi.org/10.1556/2006.5.2016.088; Advance online publication

30. Merritt A, LaQuea R, Cromwell R, Ferguson CJ. Media managing mood: a look at the possible effects of violent media on affect. Child Youth Care Forum. 2016;45:241–58. https://doi.org/10.1007/s10566-015-9328-8.
31. Johnson D, Wyeth P, Sweetser P. Creating good lives through computer games. In: Huppert FA, Cooper CL, editors. Interventions and policies to enhance wellbeing, vol. VI. Hoboken: Wiley-Blackwell; 2014. p. 485–510.
32. Durkin K. Videogames and young people with developmental disorders. Rev Gen Psychol. 2010;14(2):122–40. https://doi.org/10.1037/a0019438.
33. Olson CK. Children's motivations for video game play in the context of normal development. Rev Gen Psychol. 2010;14(2):180–7. https://doi.org/10.1007/s10964-017-0646-z.
34. Bowman ND, Kowert R, Ferguson CJ. The impact of video game play on human (and orc) development. In: Green GP, Kaufman JC, editors. Video games and creativity. San Diego: Academic Press; 2015. p. 43–58.
35. Dye M, Green C, Bavelier D. The development of attention skills in action video game players. Neuropsychologia. 2009;47(8):1780–9. https://doi.org/10.1016/j.neuropsychologia.2009(a).02.002.
36. Dye M, Green C, Bavelier D. Increasing speed of processing with action video games. Curr Dir Psychol Sci. 2009;18(6):321–6.
37. Madigan J. Forever questing and "getting gud". In: Kowert R, editor. Video games and well-being: press start. Cham: Palgrave Macmillian; 2020. p. 65–76.
38. Sherr JL. Flow and media enjoyment. Commun Theory. 2004;14:328–47.

Esports Mental Performance

8

Carl Daubert

8.1 Esports Performance Coaches

The title of "esports performance coach" is a nebulous one; its definition in esports has not been fully fleshed out or determined. A performance coach may focus on strength and conditioning or they may also focus on mental performance. Many performance coaches use a "jack-of-all-trades" approach, aiding in physical aspects like strength training and diet while also doing some work on mental techniques like mindfulness and confidence-building. This makes determining who is and is not working in the field of esports performance, in a way that is analogous to sports performance, much harder to determine. The focus of this chapter will be on mental performance and mental performance coaching for esport athletes.

The concept of auxiliary staff working with players on "softer skills" outside of practice is not new. Traditional sports have been utilizing this model for far longer. So long, in fact, that some auxiliary positions are becoming full-time careers, in large part due to their impact. Esports may be slow to adopt esports medicine, but top-tier esports organizations have quickly recognized the bene-

C. Daubert (✉)
Performance Coach Carl Consulting, Hanover Township, PA, USA

L. Migliore et al. (eds.), *Handbook of Esports Medicine*,
https://doi.org/10.1007/978-3-030-73610-1_8

fits of having coaches with varying backgrounds on staff to assist with players' needs outside of in-game mechanics and strategy. This is a significant step in the right direction since the consideration of the mental and physical well-being of esports athletes was nonexistent until recent years. However, the lack of a concrete definition for an "esports performance coach" has led to teams often being led astray. The market is flooded with well-intentioned but underqualified "performance coaches" looking to make profit in the budding industry of esports.

Esports' rapid growth has made it hard for traditional organizations like the American Psychological Association (APA) and Association for Applied Sport Psychology (AASP) to keep up with the pace. It is also difficult to create best practices when the scientific support for them is often being determined on a case-by-case basis . The path forward includes developing educational resources for organizations so they can have a better idea of what their players' needs are. This will allow for the opportunity to find qualified individuals to fill performance coaching roles. The future also includes qualified practitioners in the space joining together to dictate what ethical and quality practice looks like.

With these considerations in mind, the rest of this chapter will delve into the science of mental performance coaching in esports from the framework of sport and performance psychology. It would be improper to infer that all mental performance techniques used in traditional sport translate well to the esport population. The basis for the techniques discussed are drawn from scientific study when possible, but based on analogous population extrapolation and author experience when not.

8.2   Mental Performance Basics

When discussing the basics of mental performance, it is useful to consider first how we engage in actions by considering the self. A deeper understanding of self, known as self-awareness, is a key requirement to developing every other mental skill discussed in this section [1]. Bringing an esport athlete's attention to their thoughts and feelings requires active and deliberate training, often taking the form of journaling and individual meetings with a mental performance coach to review thoughts, feelings, and decisions made in and out of game.

Not only does the development of self-awareness allow the athlete to resolve potential problem areas dictated by their lack of self-understanding, it also gives them an excellent starting point for future mental performance training. Upon developing a moderate level of self-awareness, athletes often begin to notice how things like stress, anxiety, confidence, motivation, goal setting, and other areas within the mental performance domain can play a role in their overall ability to perform [2]. By engaging in a reciprocal and ongoing relationship with their mental performance coach, athletes are able to obtain tailored attention to ongoing needs. Applying this on a team level can also be beneficial and dictate team-building experiences that teach skills like problem-solving, anxiety management, and more.

A "needs assessment" is an excellent place for a mental performance coach to start their work with a team. Much like traditional sports, no two competitors are the same. Determining a clear picture of where each athlete stands ensures training is as effective as possible for each player. There are many considerations when doing a needs assessment that branch from in-game position to the player's age and background. This is often particularly important when athletes are playing a game with different roles. With the population of esports being so varied, cultural considerations must also be taken into account. A needs assessment is an invaluable tool and will help the practitioner determine which strategies may best fit the players' needs. An assessment can be done a variety of ways but usually entails both team and individual meetings to go over player strengths and weaknesses, as well as team cohesion and communication. Following are some of many integral pieces of a robust needs assessment.

8.2.1 Imagery

Most people have inadvertently engaged in visualization at one point or another during their lives. The vivid depiction or recollection of an event may come naturally to most people, but may be more difficult for others. When utilized, it may be to replay particularly unpleasant experiences, and seem involuntary. In that case, it may lead to increases in stress/anxiety. Where a mental performance coach can become useful is using this vivid depiction to instead imagine events of the future, and thus prepare more effectively. By imagining these scenarios as a movie, events that have yet to happen can be prepared and trained for.

By applying effort toward developing the mental skill of imagery, we can adjust the movie to play out any which way we would like. Being able to do this can have an immense positive effect on confidence, feelings of preparedness, and create reductions in pre-performance anxiety [1].

When discussing imagery, it is important to note that it is not just seeing the movie in your mind. Training the skill of imagery means trying to connect together as many senses as we possibly can. Feeling the keys under your fingertips, hearing the background music or teammate chatter through your headset, the taste of chewing gum, all these have an important place in creating a successful imagery practice.

Imagery, when done on the fly with no training, is often used by players to determine their ideal circumstances. They see how their perfect game would look and feel to them. While this may be a great way to understand the win condition of the game, taking a deliberate approach to imagery training may offer more mental flexibility. Imagery can be utilized to determine what barriers or problems a player may come across while working towards their goal. By engaging in this practice, the player may feel better prepared to manage the ever-changing circumstances in competition which will offer a potentially improved sense of confidence. The players' ability to control the mental film they are playing can give them the opportunity to see how a single situation can play out countless different ways which gives them the chance to create responses that could get them the result they are looking for.

As players develop the skill of imagery, they often become more attuned to their performances. Their ability to use their countless hours of practice will become more apparent as they recall previous gameplay moments more readily. This recollection will help strengthen the neural pathways they have constructed through practice while also allowing them to make decisions faster [3]. The basic concept of preparation boils down to repetitions done at a game-like pace; if players can utilize mental imagery effectively, they may be able to up the amount of game-like repetitions they have made which will increase their overall sense of preparation. This is also important when considering the number of ways something unexpected can happen. Players who have committed to an imagery practice are also more likely to rebound from mistakes and unexpected circumstances [3].

8.2.2 IZOF

The Individualized Zone of Optimal Functioning (IZOF) is a theory that was proposed by Juri Hanin in 1980, and has since been further developed. The theory states that every person has a certain level of arousal at which they work best. If an athlete can determine what their zone is, they can then implement training tactics to help them get into that zone as often as possible. This theoretically leads to the athlete performing at a consistently high level, which is the overall goal with most mental skills training programs. The IZOF is a fairly basic method for players to take the jitters they may feel before matches and reframe them into a useful source of energy and focus during intense moments [4].

The IZOF works on a bell curve, depicted in Fig. 8.1. The theory states that as arousal increases from rest, an athlete's ability to perform will also increase to a point. Beyond that point, athletes will start to see athletic competence decline from being over-aroused. While this is how the basic model works, it is important to note that there are individual differences that need to be taken into account when figuring out a player's IZOF. The figure below would imply that everyone works best with a moderate amount of arousal but this may not be true for everyone. There are various factors that can influence where an athlete's arousal curve fits on the plane [4].

Athletes can use their past experiences as a starting point to figure out what their bell curve may look like. Does the athlete

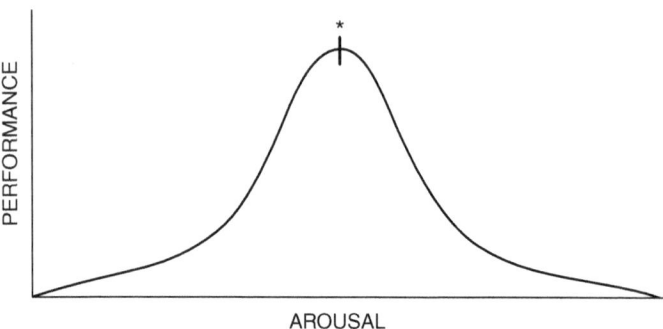

Fig. 8.1 The Individualized Zone of Optimal Functioning bell curve. The asterisk depicts the optimal arousal state of an athlete, at which point performance will theoretically be maximized

compete best in championship moments, when tension and pressure are at their highest? Do they have a history of performing at their peak in matches that "don't matter"? These are questions that can help players figure out their initial curve, though it is likely it will need tweaking and testing over time to increase accuracy. Once players have an understanding of where they exist generally on the curve, they can start to think in a more situation-specific manner. This exercise can also help determine skills the player may need to take time to develop further.

While it would be easy to assume that once an athlete finds their overall curve, they know where they need to be at all times. Unfortunately, this is rarely correct. Finding out what an athlete's general performance curve looks like is instead a starting point. Athletes will need to continue to check in and rate themselves while undergoing the variety of situations they find themselves in so they can continue to tweak the curve to suit their needs. As athletes rely on self-awareness techniques, they will be able to more readily understand their personal performance curves and thus determine what tools they need to practice to best prepare for competition.

Athletes also need to create a toolbox of mental skills to help them achieve their ideal level of arousal. An athlete who works best under lower arousal but ends up being the only player alive in a high-stakes game will want to have some arousal reduction techniques available. Similarly, a player who performs best in high-arousal environments will likely want some form of technique to increase arousal in games that are perceived as less important. Players who take the time to understand their curve and create useful techniques will increase their overall feeling of preparedness and will see the benefits of being more confident as well [4].

Coaches can play a large role in helping athletes determine their IZOF during both practice and competition. Watching their players practice and compete can give a coach a bird's-eye view to how players are reacting to fluctuations in arousal during competition. This can create helpful data for teams to use when helping athletes determine their IZOF as well as the overall team condition. This can also be an important point for coaches to keep in mind as their language (both verbal and nonverbal) can have a massive impact on a player's arousal level before, during, and after competition. A coach who can accurately find their team's IZOF will be better prepared to give them the reinforcement, and correction they need [4].

The IZOF is a great tool to help esports athletes develop a deeper understanding of how their emotional state can influence their performance. Self-awareness is crucial to any athlete looking to utilize a mental skills training program and the IZOF helps athletes develop the deeper awareness needed to start working on tangible and practical skills. While the IZOF is not the only important mental training tool, the breadth of how it can help an esport athlete makes it one of the most important to develop early on in a mental training program.

8.2.3   Confidence

Often considered the most important mental skill by esports and traditional sport athletes alike, confidence is a universally important component of being a high-performing individual. Confidence refers to a person's belief that the skill set they have can adequately meet a challenge placed in front of them [5]. Athletes often talk about confidence from a polarized point of view. They describe it as something you either have or you do not. Mental performance coaches would disagree with this assessment because confidence has been shown to be a trainable skill if you know how and are committed to deliberate practice.

Many esports athletes talk about confidence in a similar fashion to traditional sport athletes. They feel confident when they are playing their absolute best but when they are struggling, it is nowhere to be found. This is more of a "chicken-and-the egg" way of viewing confidence and actually lends itself more to the concept of self-efficacy (the belief that one can accomplish a task or goal). To handle any situation or opponent, players need confidence. From the start of the first game, players need self-efficacy to lane effectively, position well, and give accurate callouts to their teammates [2].

Self-talk is an important factor in confidence, and is often broken into positive or negative versions. The difference between the versions is self-explanatory, with positive creating confidence while negative detracts from confidence. The version a player picks is often based on an immediate risk assessment that is done when confronted with external stimuli. That is, they assess whether the knowledge and preparation they have is up to the challenge placed in front of them [3].

If a player struggles to feel confident when playing against tough opponents, it means that their risk assessment is telling them that they do not have the skill set to handle the challenge [3]. With that in mind, the challenge for a mental performance coach and the player in question becomes changing the internal narrative to more accurately reflect the reality of the situation. Some players may downplay their ability as a defense mechanism. If they lose, they may be able to deflect the negative emotions associated with loss, and may be able to manage their negative emotions better if anticipated (i.e., "Of course we lost, I knew we were going to from the minute I logged on").

Well-meaning players and performance coaches may try to use the "fake it till you make it" mantra to boost confidence when a player is not feeling confident. While this may be an effective method in the short term, it may backfire in the long run for players who never "catch up." This is similar to downplaying a match or competition's importance in order to reduce anxiety. However, it may end up creating more problems than benefits if applied long term and can very quickly turn into a loop of negative self-talk that prohibits the athlete from performing at an optimal performance level.

Interventions to help players develop a sturdy sense of confidence and self-efficacy are based around connecting practice preparation with competition. Bridges need to be built between the training and practice (in and out of game) that the player has undergone and the competitive environment in which they are being asked to work. This concept of state-dependent memory and learning can be applied in a variety of ways. The first is to practice as close to the competitive environment as possible. This will help the brain process the stress it is feeling and instead of trying to protect itself by bailing or underselling the importance, players will grow more comfortable in that environment. This is often referred to as stress inoculation [6].

Conveying the simple fact that confidence can be trained similar to mechanical skills is important for player growth. Many players base their confidence levels off of past experiences and, while our self-talk can be influenced by what has happened in the past, it is often more fragile. The method of basing confidence on preparation puts control back into the players' hands because they can control the effort and attitude they carry with them into practice. They cannot control how their last game's result went or what their opponents' future actions, but they can control their future choices. Pairing confidence with control will offer a more resilient and longer-lasting form of confidence which will help them play better consistently.

8.2.4 Goal Setting

Goal setting is a naturally occurring process that can be honed to provide performance benefits. People often consider new accomplishments or think of achievements, but the difference between the goal setting done naturally and the goal setting training done

by mental performance coaches is the systemization and utilization of scientific study to give athletes the best chance at accom-
plishing their goals. When players are left to their own devices,
they often can set goals but struggle to come up with the individual steps necessary to reach the end point.

There are two forms of goals that need to be discussed to
understand how they are used by esports athletes. The first is
external (otherwise known as product) goals. These goals are
related to a reward that the athlete will get at the end of their jour-
ney. For many professional players, this entails a championship,
MVP award, or bonus to their salary. Amateur players may have
the goal of getting onto their first professional team. High school
players may have the goal of being recruited or selected for a collegiate program. These would all be examples of external goals
because they are based on the result that the player is trying to
achieve [5].

The second form of goals are internal (otherwise known as
process) goals. These goals are based around our internal sense of
self-worth and growth. Examples of internal goals include want-
ing to get better at a certain skill set, and becoming more mindful
of one's thoughts and how they influence actions. Internal goals
provide a stronger determinant of motivation and confidence over
a longer period of time while external goals are best used in short
increments. Internal goals may be harder to create concrete steps
for and monitor progress on. This may be one reason why athletes
may set few, if any, internal goals [5].

As a person, you have complete control over two things: attitude and effort. By adjusting focus to shorter and more internal
goals, players will begin to understand the way their mindset in
the moment directly impacts their consistency. Players who are
better able to create smaller short-term goals for themselves based
around internal measures will see increase in motivation, confidence, stress/anxiety management, and other areas relating to
their performance abilities [5]. Mental performance coaches can
help esport athletes by creating measures for their internal goals
and providing them with tangible ways to monitor progress. This
can lead to more confidence, and thus increase the likelihood of
positive performance outcomes.

8.3   The Future of Esports Performance Coaching

There is not an official accreditation board currently in existence for esports performance coaching. This has led to no obvious distinction between qualified professionals and those who may lack formal training or experience. As esports continues to grow and more money is added to the equation, this problem will only worsen. To make matters worse, organizations who hire unprepared or untrained auxiliary staff may sour to the idea of any performance coach at all. They may be less likely in the future to allocate funds and time to those resources. This will subsequently hurt players and staff more than anyone else as these resources, when used correctly, not only increase performance but aid in the overall physical and mental health of players and staff.

The future of esports performance coaching is not all negative. With esports growing, practitioners from both mental and physical sides of the coaching spectrum are joining together to determine what best practices are, how to work ethically in these environments, and what they can do to continue to push the science of esports performance coaching forward for future generations.

References

1. Mack G, Casstevens D. Mind gym: an athlete's guide to inner excellence. New York: McGraw Hill; 2001.
2. Biswas-Diener R. Practicing positive psychology coaching. 1st ed. Hoboken: Wiley; 2010.
3. Taylor J. Assessment in applied sport psychology. Champaign: Human Kinetics; 2018.
4. Burton D, Raedeke TD. Sport psychology for coaches. Champaign: Human Kinetics; 2008.
5. Orlick T. In pursuit of excellence: how to win in sport and life through mental training. 5th ed. Champaign: Human Kinetics; 2016.
6. Stulburg B, Magness S. The passion paradox: a guide to going all in, finding success, and discovering the benefits of an unbalanced life. Emmaus: Rodale; 2019.

Prevention of Esports Injuries

9

Lindsey Migliore

9.1   Introduction

The tremendous growth of the esports industry in recent years has led to a disproportionate amount of players in comparison to healthcare professionals. Opportunity, in large part generated by sponsorship and investment money from companies targeting the gigantic audience, has spawned countless teams, organizations, competitions, and tournaments. As a result, an increasing number of gamers are earning sustainable livings and carving out careers for themselves as esports professionals. Yet, the healthcare industry remains relatively ignorant of the needs of this population.

The career span of a professional gamer is subjectively numbered to be between 3 and 5 years in length, although no peer-reviewed data exists on the topic. When compared to the career length seen in traditional sports where competition is arguably more physically taxing, this number pales in comparison. The reasons for this discrepancy are numerous: burnout, promotions to better paying positions, waning of a certain game title's popularity, injuries, etc. The relative lack of data on esports injuries

L. Migliore (✉)
GamerDoc, Washington, DC, USA
e-mail: doc@gamerdoc.net

213

L. Migliore et al. (eds.), *Handbook of Esports Medicine*,
https://doi.org/10.1007/978-3-030-73610-1_9

makes studying the topic frustrating; efforts by some research groups are shedding more light on the health of the esports player. Despite this, one thing is for certain: esports injuries are costly. Financially, sports-related injuries to U.S. high school and collegiate players alone costs an estimated $20 billion dollars a year [1]. Furthermore, injuries can have serious detrimental long-term health consequences, both physically and mentally.

In order to tackle this clandestine esports injury problem, a multitude of hurdles must be overcome. First, large-scale surveillance studies need to be performed to accurately assess the prevalence of injuries. Second, the mechanisms of these injuries need to be determined. Third, preventative training measures addressing these mechanisms must be designed. Fourth, these preventative measures must be studied for efficacy, implementation, and adherence. Lastly, strategies to improve adherence rates must be designed, implemented, and further studied. A seemingly gargantuan task, compounded by the relative ignorance to the field of esports medicine, and catalyzed by a culture not familiar or trusting of medical professionals, leads to the perfect storm for a brewing public health crisis.

9.1.1   The Problem of Presentation

To some, esports medicine may seem relatively redundant, or even unnecessary. Treatment of a large majority of the injuries discussed in Chaps. 2, 3, and 4 are not outside the expertise of existing sports medicine providers, or even motivated pediatricians or primary care providers. Occupational and physical therapists are trained in the rehabilitation of tenosynovitis, tendonitis, and muscular imbalances, regardless of cause. The answer is twofold. First, the esports industry does not fully recognize the prevalence and consequences of injuries. Second, gamers that do present to the aforementioned providers are often misdiagnosed and thus ineffectively treated.

9.1.2 Injury Culture

Esports arguably has an injury problem that is culturally pervasive and as ingrained into the industry as energy drinks and mechanical keyboards. There is a paucity of awareness concerning the simple fact that injuries can, and do, exist in competitive gaming. As a result, there is a general lack of emphasis on injury prevention, as one simply does not work to prevent something that does not exist. Once injured, players, coaches, and physicians are slow to attribute it to the physical act of gaming. This not only delays treatment, but often results in inaccurate diagnoses. Players are also more hesitant to seek treatment due to a multitude of causes.

The fundamental understanding of injuries can differ drastically between esports and traditional athletes due to distinctions in training history. American youth soccer begins between the ages of 3 and 5, and is a common rite of passage among those both athletically and non-athletically inclined. U.S. Soccer registers over three million children annually [2].

At this level, competition is low, and coaches are focused more on keeping children on the playing surface rather than advanced tactics. Regardless, the 40% of U.S. children who participate in sports at this age begin to learn important lessons even from this low level of participation [3].

Ankle sprains are the most common injuries in youth soccer and basketball, affecting over a third of participants [4]. These injuries can be traumatic, removing players from their sport, causing a significant amount of pain, and even requiring the use of crutches. However, ankle sprains can and do heal in the vast majority of cases. Pain abates, crutches are thrown into the far corners of the garage, and eventually a return to play occurs. This process shows athletes firsthand that *they can recover from injuries*. No matter how painful and frustrating, with medical treatment, physical therapy, and time, return to play occurs.

Esports, only recently recognized at the pediatric level as a legitimate team activity, does not have this same trajectory. Training begins in the quiet of a player's home with either one or two friends or online. Coaching at this level is relatively absent.

As players advance through the ranks, they may be invited to more advanced competitions or compete against higher level players, but remain relatively unsupervised. It is often not until a player is signed by a professional team or obtains a college scholarship that they first encounter a coach, let alone an athletic trainer. Gamers have simply not experienced the same athletic process from a young age like their traditional athletic counterparts. They have not experienced injuries related to their sport that they have been able to successfully rehabilitate, nor do they have role models or examples in the media to draw that conclusion. As a result, the majority of esports players do not fully grasp the extent of their injury, or simply *do not believe they can recover from it.*

Even once an injury is recognized, players may be hesitant to seek treatment for fear of losing their starting spots and sponsorships or risk being seen to be making excuses for declining performance. The latter is of particular importance, as performance may indeed be declining due to pain and weakness, but ignoring the issue only aggravates and accelerates the decline. Some players, like Jordan "n0thing" Gilbert, admitted to struggling with injuries, but feared going public with the implications, and chose to struggle in private. Others, like Clinton "Fear" Loomis, reportedly sought treatment after feeling symptoms only to receive an incorrect diagnosis and incorrect treatment. Barriers exist at every step of the way, even before a player steps into a doctor's office.

9.1.3   Role of the Healthcare Provider

Early in training, providers are taught the importance of taking an all-encompassing social history. Do they use alcohol or other drugs? This allows a practitioner to anticipate any drug interactions or injury susceptibilities. What is the patient's occupation? Prepatellar bursitis is an easily made diagnosis in carpet layers with knee swelling. Has the patient travelled recently to Central America? That eye swelling might not be a simple stye, but instead Chagas disease. What about gaming history? Patients presenting with wrist pain can be diagnosed, treated, and sent on their way without any mention of such. For the few providers who still ask about occupation during initial evaluations, a professional gamer may be picked up, but casual gamers are still being missed. Gaming history should become a routine line of questioning in the social history.

Additionally, once one does choose to pay attention to esports, there are further considerations. The unique challenges faced by anyone who wishes to delve into esports medicine and truly grow something from nothing are by far countered by the rewards. The earliest physicians, therapists, and trainers have the privilege of setting the tone. Traditional medicine relies heavily on post-injury treatment and interventions due to a variety of factors with which anyone who does their own charting and billing is all too familiar. Esports medicine, however, can be based on prevention.

9.2 The Impact of Injury

When evaluating the true impact of competitive injuries, not only must the negative consequences be discussed, but also the absence of the positive benefits of esports participation. Involvement in both traditional sports and esports can have profound implications to a player's life. While researchers have found varying and often contradictory effects of video games on academic performance, esports participation resoundingly improves academics [5, 6]. High school esports involvement was associated with improved graduation rates and increased GPAs [7].

The outcropping of high school and collegiate esports teams results in the overall growth of STEM programs and drives recruitment. However, unlike traditional athletics regulated by the NCAA, there is no centralized governance. As a result, health screenings are not required and athletics department involvement is school-specific (and usually absent). At the professional level, esports players, despite using their bodies to perform competitively, are not classified as athletes but rather as "talent." Therefore, organizations and teams cannot require medical evaluations or treatment of their players. Furthermore, the providers knowledgeable about esports medicine are sparse, leading to a barrier to treatment even if treatment were desired.

Despite this, esports injuries are occurring and resulting in missed competitions, declining performance, and even quitting entirely. Early studies on the incidence of esports injuries largely focus on collegiate teams. Very little is known about the plight of professional players, as speaking publicly can threaten their hard-earned spot or be made to be seen as an "excuse" for poor performance. Athletes usually only speak up after they are forced into an early retirement, and use nonofficial platforms such as Reddit or social media. Players who have spoken publicly about their injuries and the detrimental effects it has had on their careers are shown in Table 9.1. As a result, esports athletes who suffer an

Table 9.1 Esports athletes who have spoken publicly about injuries and the impact on their careers

Name	Game	Injury	Impact
Toyz	League of Legends	Carpal tunnel syndrome	Initial retirement at 21
Hai	League of legends	Wrist	Initial retirement at 22
Uzi	League of Legends	Arm	Retirement at 23
TheShy	League of Legends	Wrist	Missed competitions
Flash	StarCraft	Arm	Missed competitions
Fear	Dota 2	Radial nerve	Initial retirement at 26
ZooMaa	Call of Duty	Thumb	Initial retirement at 25
Olofmeister	Counter-Strike	Hand	Missed competitions
Freeze	League of Legends	Wrist tendonitis	Missed competitions
Mantuu	Counter-Strike	DeQuervain's tenosynovitis	Missed competitions
Issa	Fortnite	Carpal tunnel syndrome	Retirement at 19
GuardiaN	Counter-Strike	Carpal tunnel syndrome	Missed competitions

injury are seemingly less likely to seek treatment, and suffer the financial, mental, and physical consequences of such without effective support.

Of note, players often initially retired due to injuries, and then returned to play after extended rehabilitation and interventions.

9.2.1 Financial Consequences

Traditional sports injuries are so pervasive and financially detrimental that they are considered a public health concern. Therefore, a significant amount of scientific and medical resources have been devoted to averting these. Effective sports injury prevention programs have been shown to save systems millions of dollars [1].

For traditional sports athletes, injuries can have catastrophic effects not only on their mental well-being, but career span and earnings. National Football League players with ACL tears had shorter career spans when compared to their uninjured teammates, and earned two million dollars less in salary [8].

For esports players, injuries do not exist in a vacuum. Wrist pain, leading to an inability to perform while gaming will also affect other facets of life. While some professional players can earn a comfortable living from solely gaming, high school, collegiate, and amateur athletes must go to school or jobs. Declines in school and job performance have yet to be studied in this population after injury, but one can reasonably infer correlation if not causation.

Organizations who have invested countless amounts of money and time into player development are left with players performing at less than peak or sitting on the sidelines. This comparison can directly be carried over into esports. Player development can take months and years. Delicate team compositions focused on player roles, such as an effective top-laner in multiplayer online battle arena (MOBA) games or support players in titles like Overwatch or Valorant, can be decimated by the loss of one individual. Unlike traditional sports, where advanced rehabilitation teams can use mechanisms and technology unavailable to the regular public, rehabilitation for esports injuries is relatively nonexistent. Injuries can, and have, ended professional esports careers with no return to play. This results in financial loss for both the player and the organization.

9.2.2 Physical Health Complications

While the long-term consequences of esports injuries are unknown and will likely not be discovered for years, data can be extrapolated from the existing literature. Until long-term studies are performed on esports athletes, the following complications are purely speculative and should be treated as such. Diagnosticians are encouraged to rely on existing data, and when that data is nonexistent, epistemic curiosity.

9.2.2.1 Acute Tendon Injuries

A large majority of esports injuries are the result of repetitive movements resulting in chronic tendinopathy. Pathological tendon, its architecture fundamentally altered due to years of misuse, is more susceptible to an acute injury, whether that is during or outside of gaming [9, 10]. Mouse and keyboard players with smoldering extensor carpi ulnaris (ECU) tendinopathy may not feel any pain while gaming, but suffer an acute ECU injury during an unrelated activity, such as a morale-boosting bowling night. The weakened tendon tears under the weight of the bowling ball and improper form, causing an acute or chronic injury. However, the player felt the pain when bowling, so does not attribute the injury to gaming. This further compounds diagnosis and may lead to improper treatment.

9.2.2.2 Osteoarthritis

Osteoarthritis (OA) results from the degeneration of joint cartilage, leading to underlying bone damage. Causes of primary arthritis include obesity, alteration in sex hormone levels, occupational risk factors (such as repetitive lifting or climbing), and joint damage [11].

Joint injury is the leading cause of early post-traumatic OA, with an estimated fourfold increase of developing OA following knee joint injury [12]. Athletes are more likely to sustain a joint injury when compared to non-athletes. Subsequently, elite athletes in high-contact sports have a higher risk of developing knee and hip arthritis later in life than non-athletes [13]. However, a majority of these cases deal with lower extremity OA in large, weight-bearing joints, something that would logically not be related to esports. Increased rates of hand and wrist OA, however, have been correlated previously with repetitive use [14].

Trapeziometacarpal joint (TMJ), also known as the carpometacarpal joint, is the second most common hand joint affected by osteoarthritis, and can have a profound impact on function [15]. Due to the biconcave-convex saddle joint structure, the TMJ relies on surrounding ligaments for stability. This can place the joint under incredible pressures, further increased by ligamentous dysfunction. Repetitive use can accelerate TMJ wear and tear, as well as resulting disability [14].

Additionally, a majority of gamers are still in development and have not yet reached skeletal maturity. Overuse can lead to physeal injuries, and thus irreversible damage to growing cells. The weakest physiologic structure of the bone in the pediatric population, damage to the physis can result in growth disturbances. These effects have been well-documented in traditional pediatric athletes [16].

9.3   Understanding Esports Injuries

Esports injuries occur and can have a profound impact on multiple facets of a player's life as well as their team and organization. So the question then becomes, how can this issue be effectively and scientifically addressed? Not only must this question be answered, but in order for true systemic change to occur, it must be universally applicable to all esports athletes, readily and easily adoptable by teams and organizations, and continuously studied and improved. Luckily, this question has been tackled long ago by traditional sports.

9.3.1   Fatigue

Neuromuscular fatigue, caused by extensive and prolonged gaming sessions, is an important target for any injury prevention program. Effectively addressing fatigue when it occurs can, not only prevent injury, but represent an interesting performance paradigm, as training to resist fatigue can reduce injury incidence [17].

9.3.1.1   Causes of Fatigue

A fatigued muscle has a decreased maximal force when compared to non-fatigued muscle, which results from a variety of peripheral and central mechanisms [18, 19].

Peripheral fatigue mechanisms result from a decrease in force-generating capacity of the muscle. Intramuscularly, decreased contractile forces generally result when substrates for ATP generation are depleted or when accumulation of by-products that interfere with contractibility. Once immediate sources of energy are used, glycogen is used for metabolism producing lactic acid. The relative acidity of the muscle then increases, further negatively affecting performance.

Central fatigue is thought to stem for a reduction in the level of voluntary muscle activation. Decreased motor unit firing rates have been observed with isometric loading. Central fatigue is thought to be more pronounced during submaximal exercise activity, which is more relevant to the esports population [18].

9.3.1.2   Effect of Fatigue

Neuromuscular fatigue, via both peripheral and central causes, can have profound health and performance consequences. Anterior cruciate ligament (ACL) tears, one of the most common injuries in traditional sports, occur primarily during noncontact plays. Multiple studies have implicated fatigue-induced altered biomechanics as the underlying cause of this phenomenon. Muscle fatigue provides decreased active joint stabilization, drastically affecting ACL loads [18].

Furthermore, fatigued muscle can have notable effects outside of the immediate environment by affecting biomechanics and proprioception. Muscle fatigue has also been shown to be correlated with decreased velocity of movement and accuracy [20, 21]. In overhead throwing, functional fatigue affects the entire upper extremity – not just muscles directly involved [22]. The entire kinetic chain is altered due to adjusted biomechanics. Altered biomechanics place more distal joints under increased stress, thus increasing the risk of potential injury. With prolonged throws, pitchers threw lower-velocity pitches and experienced more pain.

Pitching fatigue resulted in increased torque on the medial elbow, a risk factor for ulnar collateral (UCL) tears [23].

As fatigue worsened, muscles more distal began to exert more influence. As more pitches were thrown, prior to changes noticed in upper extremity kinetics, core and leg musculature also experienced fatigue. Therefore, core and leg strengthening may also serve as training targets [24].

These findings, coupled with the effect that core musculature can exert on back pain, suggest that core training may serve as an interesting and beneficial target for esports athletes.

9.3.1.3 Fatigue Protocols

Fatigue protocols, or sets of exercises designed to simulate sports-specific fatigue, have been developed for traditional sports. These protocols are designed to decrease muscle force production and decay proprioception to simulate real life, in-game fatigue. Using these protocols, the behavior of joints and extremities can be studied under fatigue for altered biomechanics [25].

For example, unilateral leg fatigue has been shown to result in altered knee and hip angles, placing more stress on ligaments like the ACL [21]. Athletic trainers and therapists utilize these fatigue protocols to evaluate their athletes and subsequent susceptibility to ACL tears. This allows them to address risk factors via tailored training programs, thus preventing these injuries before they occur.

The development of fatigue protocols can inform sports-specific training programs by identifying common areas of susceptibility, and implement flexibility and strengthening paradigms. To date, there is no data on the effect of neuromuscular fatigue on the esports athlete. The central question of "does gaming fatigue affect biomechanics?" is virtually impossible to answer as we know very little about the "normal" biomechanics of esports.

9.3.2   Biomechanics and Biodynamics of Esports

Each athletic movement is a summation of its parts. A quarterback's throw is a result of the placement of her feet on the ground, angle of the ankles, bend of the knees, loading of the lower limbs, limits of hip rotation, core strength, shoulder girdle stabilization, and loading of her throwing arm. The force generated by the arm resulting in a throw is generated by factors much more distal. For high-performing athletes, each individual constituent can be optimized to not only prevent injuries resulting from improper or inefficient biomechanics, but improve throwing accuracy and speed. While force may not be a desired result in esports, accuracy certainly is desirable.

While, for football, outside of the 2014 American Football Conference Championship game, the ball size and shape do not change, esports does not have such luxury. Competitive gaming takes place on a variety of inputs, including but not limited to: mouse and keyboard, console controllers, and arcade sticks. The biomechanics of playing, essentially how a player controls their movements, has not been scientifically studied.

The most commonly utilized input, mouse and keyboard, has even more variability depending on the gaming title. MOBA games utilize a combination of keyboard inputs with mouse movement. Traditional FPS games like Call of Duty or Valorant utilize WASD directional keybinds with one hand, while the other utilizes a mouse for complex movements coordinating aim. Games with more complicated keyboard mechanics, such as building in Fortnite, place varying levels of stress on both extremities depending on the in-game situation.

Mouse movement varies by person. Players may rely on either their wrist radial and ulnar deviation or shoulder flexion/abduction primarily for large motions. Every joint of the upper extremity is involved. For a right-handed mouse player, to target left, players may utilize radial deviation, pronation, elbow flexion, shoulder internal rotation, flexion, or extension (amongst other movements). Constant contraction of the shoulder stabilizers maintains accuracy and precision, as well mouse grip via hand and wrist muscles.

This information is based primarily on experience and speculation, with no research-based, nerve conduction or electromyography studies to draw upon. Furthermore, to what degree a player utilizes these motions is based upon a plethora of other factors (e.g., sensitivity, mouse counts per inch (CPI), specific game, and in-game role). Console players, long ignored by "serious" esports titles, differ entirely, relying more heavily on forearm stabilizers and thumb muscles. To establish baseline esports biomechanics, researchers must observe esports athletes in their native setups, preferably with the assistance of trained kinesiologists.

9.3.3   Development of Esports-Specific Fatigue Protocols

Once the kinesiology of an esports athlete is more closely understood, researchers can then study this under fatigue.

Esports-specific fatigue protocols can only be established after baseline biomechanics are understood. This will allow researchers to determine the effect fatigue can have on said movements. As anticipated, fatigue protocols will differ widely between titles. StarCraft, a real-time strategy (RTS) game with some of the highest recorded actions per minute, focuses on excessive, often repetitive keyboard inputs. The keyboard hand is thus placed under differing levels of tension and stress than other titles. In order to be successful in StarCraft, players must have a higher fatigue tolerance for their keyboard hand than other titles.

After esports-specific fatigue protocols have been developed, the effect of prolonged gaming on biomechanics can be studied in a reliable manner. Although a seemingly daunting task given the body of work and the amount of competitive gaming titles, the concept of aim provides an interesting initial step towards understanding the effect fatigue can have on injury propensity.

Across most titles, the ability to accurately place your reticle or cursor on the correct target is correlated with success and skill. Thus, the authors propose those who wish to tackle this daunting topic start with fatigue protocols for aiming in both PC and console gaming. Accuracy and precision are easily quantifiable with the advent of advanced programs such as AimLab, and can be studied across a variety of environments.

Simple designs that track aim performance and decay with fatigue, as well as recovery after varying bouts of rest, can have far-reaching and more complex implications than their initial purpose. However, these studies must not fall into the same inherent flaws that others have by focusing only on one demographic, as there are documented differences in muscle fatigue between genders and other categories [26].

9.3.4   Injury Prevention Model Development

As integral as fatigue-protocols have been in helping combat ACL tears, effective esports fatigue protocols can start to inform specific risk factors to injury, and thus design interventions to address those.

9.3.4.1 van Mechelen Model

The foundation of traditional sports models is based on the work of van Mechelen [27]. This four-step model calls for the development of these programs based primarily on epidemiological research. Population surveillance is conducted to determine the exact extent of an injury. Soccer players suffer from ankle sprains, knee injuries, and Achilles tendonitis. Football players are more susceptible to ACL tears and cartilage injuries. Volleyball leads to more finger tendon disruptions. These statements are based on large studies examining emergency room visits, and have sample sizes in the millions [28].

Once injury type is established, the mechanism of injury must be determined. How do the large majority of these injuries occur? Basketball players suffer injuries when they land from a jump, football players during contact. Once that question is answered, measures can be developed to target that specific mechanism. Will high-top basketball shoes or preventative ankle braces decrease the risk of ankle sprains? After that, the population must then again be surveyed to determine if the preventative measures are successful. High-top shoes and ankle bracing do not decrease the risk of first-time ankle sprains, but bracing may prevent repeat injury [29, 30].

The current state of esports research has barely broached step one. Case studies have been performed on the incidence and prevalence of injuries, but are lacking in terms of population size and diversity of demographic. The first step to implementing effective injury prevention protocols in esports is to determine exactly what injuries are being experienced. This must be done, not only globally, but by game title, and PC versus console. Risk factors to injury, such as keyboard style and orientation, mouse size, chair, etc. must be determined and included in these studies. Using the data, injury prevention strategies can be developed and implemented. Once implemented, ongoing population surveillance must be conducted to determine efficacy.

9.3.4.2 Translating Research into the Injury Prevention Practice Framework

Early critics of van Mechelen's techniques stated the model was too academic, and did not factor in the extent to which a program was adaptable. For example, an injury prevention model that seeks to decrease the risk of ankle sprains by placing athletes in cryotherapy chambers after practice may, in theory, work. However, this is impractical for a large majority of athletes who do not have access to such equipment.

As a result, the Translating Research into the Injury Prevention Practice (TRIPP) Framework was built upon van Mechelen's paradigm by two additional steps to focus more on programs that were implementable, and not just the best scientifically or academically, as shown in Fig. 9.1 [31].

TRIPP considers factors that might impair implementation, such as player age, level, and organization. This allows for an extra understanding of the real world for which that program is being developed. Utilizing the TRIPP framework, esports injury prevention protocols must be able to generate buy-in from not

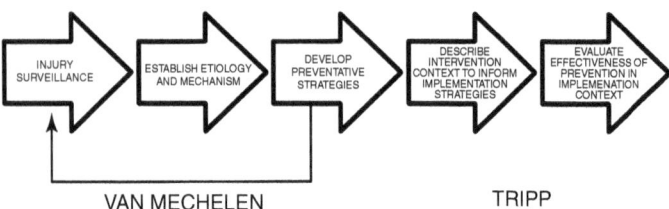

Fig. 9.1 The van Mechelen and Translating Research into the Injury Prevention Practice (TRIPP). Frameworks of developing sports injury prevention models. The TRIPP model extends upon its predecessor with two additional steps

only players, but coaches, teams, and esports organizations. Extensive warm-up routines, or exercises that require moving from the gaming setup will simply not be utilized, and thus deemed worthless. What will esports athletes do? What will not they do? These are the questions the TRIPP framework considers, where van Mechelen did not.

9.3.4.3 Reach Efficacy Adoption Implementation Maintenance Framework

The Reach Efficacy Adoption Implementation Maintenance (RE-AIM) framework was developed in team ball sports, by the creator of the TRIPP model [32]. Like its predecessor, it focuses further on the reach of the intervention, factoring in real-life application. RE-AIM goes even further to factor in the cost of a program and maintenance over time.

Widely accepted traditional sports injury prevention programs are based on these frameworks. Similarly, utilizing these frameworks, esports injury prevention programs can be designed that are not only theoretically effective, but adaptable and reproducible.

9.4   Sports Injury Prevention Models

Traditional, accepted models of sports injury prevention are based on three areas: training, rule modification, and equipment recommendations. None of these categories exist in a vacuum and improvements in one can have drastic impacts on the others. These categories tackle both intrinsic, meaning athlete-related factors, as well as extrinsic, environmental concerns. Youth hockey injuries can be confronted by looking at athlete strength, flexibility, endurance and balance, as well as rules that can be instituted to prevent injury and equipment improvements that can protect better.

9.4.1 Training

Traditional training strategies focus on addressing flexibility, strength, range of motion, endurance, and balance. These are modifiable risk factors, meaning they can be addressed with a properly designed program. Biomechanical factors, such as posture and alignment are just as important as neuromuscular factors such as strength. In fact, strength training alone has no effect on injury rates when used in isolation [33].

Neuromuscular training programs have curried favor for their ability to address all of these factors and have been found to lower the risk of musculoskeletal injuries by over 35% [34]. This model focuses on functional stability and quality of movement, which allows it to have more real-world implications. These programs are focused on agility, balance, and strength, and include levels of progression that can be tailored to different levels of athlete.

The most successful programs are multifaceted, addressing all modifiable risk factors that may increase the risk of injury. Factoring in the lessons taught by the RE-AIM framework, above all else, training programs must be realistic, be easy to integrate into normal routine, and require no special equipment [35].

9.4.1.1 Flexibility and Stretching

Stretching has long been the topic of research and point of contention for injury-prevention experts. Contrary to what the majority of the population believes, stretching before exercise has not been shown to reduce the risk of injury [36, 37]. However, improved joint flexibility can have profound implications not so simply ignored. Increased muscle flexibility allows for extended ranges of motion, decreased pain, and increased resistance to muscle injuries. This becomes even more important for esports athletes, as range of motion may be far from anatomical.

Joint range of motion is dictated by both the structure of the joint itself and the surrounding musculature. With the latter in a state of increased tension from years of negligence and overuse, addressing muscle flexibility can restore normal range of motion. This will allow players to improve their mobility, strength, and performance.

Stretching to maintain and improve flexibility is an important component of all injury prevention programs. However, the type of stretching required varies depending on the circumstances. There are multiple types of stretching, with the three most commonly used categories being static, dynamic, and pre-contraction stretching. All three result in increased range of motion, but have different effects [37].

Static Stretching

Static stretching is defined as "controlled continuous movement to end range of motion of a single joint" [38].

A static stretch is held in the lengthened position for a period of time. Experts agree that static stretching should **not** be performed prior to competition or exercise, as it may decrease muscle strength and power, theoretically increasing the risk of injury. This phenomenon has been deemed a "stretch-induced strength loss." Further study found that stretches held for less than 60 s may only have a trivial and temporary negative effect that would only be felt by high-level athletes. However, as a precaution, static stretching should not be used before exercise, but rather after to aid recovery [39].

Dynamic Stretching

Dynamic stretching can be divided into active or ballistic. Active dynamic stretching involves moving a joint through it full range of motion multiple times. As opposed to static stretching, less emphasis is placed upon maintaining the muscle in its lengthened position. Ballistic stretching, out of favor due to the increased risk of injury, involves "bouncing" at the end range [37].

Active, dynamic stretching has been shown to improve performance facets such as agility, speed, and strength. As a result, dynamic stretching is preferred to static prior to exercise [40].

Pre-contraction Stretching

The most utilized form of pre-contraction stretching is proprioceptive neuromuscular facilitation (PNF) stretching. PNF is more commonly utilized than consciously appreciated, and involves the contraction of a stretched muscle, or its antagonist. PNF recruits the Golgi tendon reflex, which results in an inhibitory effect on the contracting muscle. Designed as a protective mechanism to prevent dangerous levels of tension, it can accentuate the benefit of an individual stretch and result in a greater range of motion than a static stretch alone [41].

9.4.1.2 Strengthening

Strengthening exercises, used in conjunction with other techniques, can have a significant impact on rates of injury. Muscles with increased strength are more adept at maintaining joint stability and proper biomechanics. Rather than just grossly strengthening, effective strength training programs address specific muscle imbalances and may address areas of relative weakness that can predispose to injury. Hamstring injuries are common in running sports and can have significant performance consequences, extended return to play times, and high rates of reinjury. Strengthening programs targeting eccentric knee flexor conditioning have shown to reduce risks of hamstring strain injury [42, 43]. Different protocols might also utilize different types of muscle contraction, either concentric, isometric, and eccentric.

Concentric

Concentric muscle contraction is the most commonly understood among the general public, and incorporates providing resistance to a contracting muscle. An example of this is flexing the elbow during a bicep curl to train the biceps brachii. Concentric contraction is effective in building muscle and strength, but may place joints under more stress than other forms of contraction.

Isometric

Isometric muscle contraction occurs when a muscle is contracted, but there is no visible movement. Examples include holding a weight in a stationary position or a plank pose. Isometric protocols are often instituted acutely post-injury or in patients with underlying osteoarthritis, as they result in decreased pain when compared to other modalities.

Eccentric

Eccentric muscle contraction introduces resistance to a lengthening muscle (the opposite of concentric). The eccentric phase of a bicep curl is lowering the weight during elbow extension with the biceps brachii lengthening. Eccentric contraction generates the greatest forces when compared to other contraction types, and consumes less oxygen and energy than its concentric counterpart [44].

This phase of contraction is often ignored but provides some of the most exciting training considerations. Muscle injury and soreness are more common with eccentric contraction, but result in greater gains in strength [45].

Eccentric contraction leads to the greatest degree of delayed onset muscle soreness (DOMS), which is felt 24–72 h after exercise and results from microtrauma to muscle fibers. Receptive eccentric exercise reduces this effect, and a small amount of low intensity exercise to the region of soreness can reduce symptoms. Eccentric contractions are often the cause of muscle injury, but eccentric training can decrease muscle vulnerability to this mechanism of injury [46]. Any training program utilizing eccentric muscle contraction must lead with caution and be implemented slower to prevent both injury and soreness-related lapses in adherence.

9.4.1.3 Additional Considerations

While esports can model some of its protocols off traditional sports, factors like aerobic fitness capacity and balance may have a varying, and lesser, importance. However, core stability and muscular endurance are important considerations. Core stability itself can have a profound effect on lower and upper extremity movement. A decrease in core strength can have a negative influence on shoulder strength [47]. Furthermore, core strengthening can have a profound impact on back health, as discussed in Chap. 3.

Similarly, postural issues can be addressed via training and with ergonomic modifications. The ergonomics of esports is discussed at length in Chap. 5. Other factors, such as periodization of training and load modification, can also have important training significance but are outside of the scope of this text.

9.4.2 Rule Modification

The responsibility of injury prevention does lie solely with the athlete, and also the organizational structures creating and enforcing rules. Organizations and governing bodies can take a great deal of ownership in preventing injuries, and there are multiple examples of rule modifications in traditional sports that have resulted in a decreased rate of injury.

Starting in the 2013 season, Hockey Canada delayed allowable body checking until the Bantam division (ages 13–14) in an effort to combat concussions. This was based on multiple systematic reviews that found Pee Wee leagues (ages 11–12) who allowed body checking had a two to fourfold increase in injury when compared with non-body checking leagues. As a direct result of this rule change, there was a 50% reduction in injuries and a 64% reduction in concussion rates in Pee Wee hockey players [48]. Similarly, rugby and American football leagues have instituted tackling rules to prevent rates of concussion and injury with similar successes [49].

While rates of acute, traumatic injuries and concussion are almost negligible in esports, this idea can easily be extrapolated. Tournaments and leagues can control the length of play by adjusting the number of matches per competition. Teams can institute practice length limits and mandate ergonomic adjustments. However, changes should be based on research-backed and established risk factors and not simple speculation.

9.4.3 Equipment Recommendations

The institution of protective equipment has had a significant hand of lowering rates of injuries in multiple sports. Ankle sprains, one of the most common injuries in multiple sports, can increase the risk of re-injury by affecting ligament laxity and other supporting structures. Athletes who experience one ankle sprain are more likely than their non-injured peers to experience reinjury. Preventative ankle-taping and ankle-bracing can reduce the risk of reinjury by 70% [50]. Similarly, wrist guards utilized by snowboarders can reduce the risk of injuries such as fracture and sprains when compared to no protective gear [51].

Equipment and rule modifications are often instituted alongside significant public backlash. New cricket helmet regulations designed to reduce the risk of head injuries were ridiculed due to the effect on batting vision. Hockey cages designed to protect the face are still not utilized by professional players. In American football, helmet-to-helmet penalty calls (instituted to decrease the risk of head and neck injuries) that result in player ejections are common topics of discussion and often ridiculed.

Any modifications made to esports play are likely to come with significant backlash. Hence, it must be stressed that all recommendations must be based on a growing body of evidence and factor in other methods that might lead to institution.

9.5 Implementation and Adherence

Injury prevention programs can and do work if a few simple rules are followed. Implementation practices must be carefully crafted to ensure a well-designed program can be effective. First and foremost, medical professionals need to be involved in every single esports organization that wishes to compete at the highest level. Furthermore, *they must have influence.* Involving physicians and trainers to simply "check a box" of health and wellness is not sufficient [52].

Second, coaches and staff members must be educated and involved in training protocols. The hierarchy of responsibility must also be considered. In traditional sports programs, the lowest level of responsibility belongs with the child and the highest level on organizations or groups [34]. In an esports context, that means placing the burden on teams and organizations rather than the individual athlete.

Adherence, defined as "the extent to which a person's behavior, taking medication, following a diet, and/or executing lifestyle changes, corresponds with agreed recommendations from a health care provider" has long plagued the medical community since the advent of the profession [53].

Learned more recently by providers who chose to write a prescription for opioids rather than addressing lifestyle, weight, and biomechanics, what is done in the office can have far-reaching consequences. Despite providing irrefutable evidence towards the benefit of an intervention, unless it is adoptable, it will be ineffective.

Owoeye developed a four-step approach towards promoting adherence to an intervention, as shown in Fig. 9.2 [4]. This encourages researchers to study the rate of adherence after a prevention program is instituted, as well as identify any modifications individuals are utilizing. From there, predictors of nonadherence can be identified, and determined if they are program-based, psychosocial, club-based, socioeconomic, etc. These factors can then be addressed via strategies designed to target adherence, and these strategies are then subsequently implemented. From there, the process is repeated to study how these implementations affected adherence.

Lastly, but certainly not least, parents must be closely included for gamers. Obviously, parental permission is required for any intervention, but it must go beyond that. Parents need to be educated, not only on esports in general, but the injuries their child may be susceptible to and what they can do to prevent this. It is only with a combination of all of these factors, and likely more that the authors have not identified, that effective injury prevention protocols can take shape.

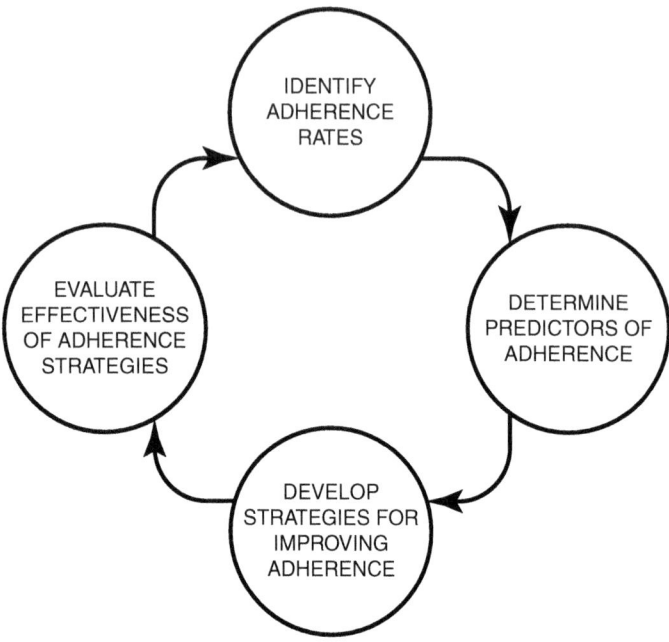

Fig. 9.2 Owoeye's four-step approach towards promoting adherence of injury prevention protocols [4]

9.6   Final Thoughts

While esports can take lessons and pages out of traditional sports' playbook, we must not fall victim to the same mistakes. Over a third of esports athletes identify as women [54]. The vast majority of early sports injury prevention studies were performed primarily on men. Textbooks often relegate women to a separate chapter under "special considerations." Furthermore, significant efforts must be made to include diverse demographics in these studies. We must aim to determine the injury propensity of esports athletes, and not just white, male esports athletes.

References

1. Fair RC, Champa C. Estimated costs of contact in college and high school male sports. J Sports Econ. 2018;20:690–717.
2. Who is US Youth Soccer? In: US Youth Soccer. https://www.usyouthsoccer.org/about/who-is-us-youth-soccer/#:~:text=US%20Youth%20Soccer%20registers%20nearly,million%20administrators%2C%20coaches%20and%20volunteers. Accessed 1 Mar 2021.
3. State of play: trends and developments in youth Sports. The Aspen Institute; 2019. https://www.aspeninstitute.org/publications/state-of-play-2019-trends-and-developments. Accessed 2 Feb 2021.
4. Owoeye OB, Palacios-Derflingher LM, Emery CA. Prevention of ankle sprain injuries in youth soccer and basketball: effectiveness of a neuromuscular training program and examining risk factors. Clin J Sport Med. 2018;28:325–31.
5. Wright J. The effects of video game play on academic performance. PsycEXTRA Dataset. 2011; https://doi.org/10.1037/e568882012-005.
6. Drummond A, Sauer JD. Video-games do not negatively impact adolescent academic performance in science, mathematics or reading. PLoS ONE. 2014; https://doi.org/10.1371/journal.pone.0087943.
7. The state of NJCAA Esports: program trends & data-drive approach to program creation. NJCAA; 2020. https://www.linkedin.com/posts/alex-mcneil_njcaae-esports-data-activity-6691844820853379072-uvFM/.
8. Secrist ES, Bhat SB, Dodson CC. The financial and professional impact of anterior cruciate ligament injuries in National Football League athletes. Orthop J Sports Med. 2016;4:232596711666392.
9. Dean BJF, Dakin SG, Millar NL, Carr AJ. Review: emerging concepts in the pathogenesis of tendinopathy. Surgeon. 2017;15:349–54.
10. Rees JD, Wilson AM, Wolman RL. Current concepts in the management of tendon disorders. Rheumatology. 2016;45:508–21.
11. Swedish Council on Health Technology Assessment. Occupational exposures and osteoarthritis: a systematic review and assessment of medical, social and ethical aspects. Stockholm: Swedish Council on Health Technology Assessment; 2016. https://www.ncbi.nlm.nih.gov/books/NBK448034/.
12. Richmond SA, Fukuchi RK, Ezzat A, Schneider K, Schneider G, Emery CA. Are joint injury, sport activity, physical activity, obesity, or occupational activities predictors for osteoarthritis? A systematic review. J Orthop Sports Phys Ther. 2013; https://doi.org/10.2519/jospt.2013.4796.
13. Tveit M, Rosengren BE, Nilsson JÅ, Karlsson MK. Former male elite athletes have a higher prevalence of osteoarthritis and arthroplasty in the hip and knee than expected. Am J Sports Med. 2012;40(3):527–33.

14. Batra S, Kanvinde R. Osteoarthritis of the thumb trapeziometacarpal joint. Curr Orthop. 2007;21:135–44.
15. Nicholas RM, Calderwood JW. De la Caffiniere arthroplasty for basal thumb joint osteoarthritis. J Bone Joint Surg Br. 1992;74-B:309–12.
16. Arnold A, Thigpen CA, Beattie PF, Kissenberth MJ, Shanley E. Overuse physeal injuries in youth athletes. Sports Health. 2017;9:139–47.
17. Quammen D, Cortes N, Van Lunen BL, Lucci S, Ringleb SI, Onate J. Two different fatigue protocols and lower extremity motion patterns during a stop-jump task. J Athl Train. 2012;47:32–41.
18. Gandevia SC. Spinal and supraspinal factors in human muscle fatigue. Physiol Rev. 2001;81:1725–89.
19. Mair SD, Seaber AV, Glisson RR, Garrett WE. The role of fatigue in susceptibility to acute muscle strain injury. Am J Sports Med. 1996;24:137–43.
20. Freeston J, Adams R, Ferdinands RED, Rooney K. Indicators of throwing arm fatigue in elite adolescent male baseball players. J Strength Cond Res. 2014;28:2115–20.
21. Mclean SG, Samorezov J. Fatigue-induced ACL injury risk stems from a degradation in central control. Med Sci Sports Exerc. 2019;41:1661–72.
22. Tripp BL, Yochem EM, Uhl TL. Functional fatigue and upper extremity sensorimotor system acuity in baseball athletes. J Athl Train. 2007;42(1):90–8.
23. Okoroha KR, Meldau JE, Lizzio VA, Meta F, Stephens JP, Moutzouros V, Makhni EC. Effect of fatigue on medial elbow torque in baseball pitchers: a simulated game analysis. Am J Sports Med. 2018;46:2509–13.
24. Erickson BJ, Sgori T, Chalmers PN, Vignona P, Lesniak M, Bush-Joseph CA, Verma NN, Romeo AA. The impact of fatigue on baseball pitching mechanics in adolescent male pitchers. Arthroscopy. 2016;32:762–71.
25. Jildeh TR, Okoroha KR, Tramer JS, Chahla J, Nwachukwu BU, Annin S, Moutzouros V, Bush-Joseph C, Verma N. Effect of fatigue protocols on upper extremity neuromuscular function and implications for ulnar collateral ligament injury prevention. Orthop J Sports Med. 2019;7:232596711988887.
26. Salomoni S, Soares FA, de Oliveira Nascimento FA, da Rocha AF. Gender differences in muscle fatigue of the biceps brachii and influences of female menstrual cycle in electromyography variables. 2008 30th Annual international conference of the IEEE Engineering in Medicine and Biology Society. 2018; https://doi.org/10.1109/iembs.2008.4649732.
27. van Mechelen W, Hlobil H, Kemper HCG. Incidence, severity, aetiology and prevention of sports injuries. Sports Med. 1992;14:82–99.
28. Mills A, Rutherford G, Marcy N. Hazard screening report: team sports: Consumer Product Safety Commission; 2004. https://www.cpsc.gov/Research%2D%2DStatistics/Sports%2D%2DRecreation.
29. McKay GD. Ankle injuries in basketball: injury rate and risk factors. Br J Sports Med. 2001;35:103–8.

30. Vuurberg G, Hoorntje A, Wink LM, van der Doelen BFW, van den Bekerom MP, Dekker R, van Dijk CN, Krips R, Loogman MCM, Ridderikhof ML, Smithuis FF, Stufkens SAS, Verhagen EALM, de Bie RA, Kerkhoffs GMMJ. Diagnosis, treatment and prevention of ankle sprains: update of an evidence-based clinical guideline. Br J Sports Med. 2018; https://doi.org/10.1136/bjsports-2017-098106. Epub 2018 Mar 7.
31. Finch C. A new framework for research leading to sports injury prevention. J Sci Med Sport. 2006;9:3–9.
32. O'Brien J, Finch CF. The implementation of musculoskeletal injury-prevention exercise programmes in team ball sports: a systematic review employing the RE-AIM framework. Sports Med. 2014;44:1305–18.
33. Herman DC, Oñate JA, Weinhold PS, Guskiewicz KM, Garrett WE, Yu B, Padua DA. The effects of feedback with and without strength training on lower extremity biomechanics. Am J Sports Med. 2009;37:1301–8.
34. Emery CA, Roy T-O, Whittaker JL, Nettel-Aguirre A, van Mechelen W. Neuromuscular training injury prevention strategies in youth sport: a systematic review and meta-analysis. Br J Sports Med. 2015;49:865–70.
35. Lauersen JB, Bertelsen DM, Andersen LB. The effectiveness of exercise interventions to prevent sports injuries: a systematic review and meta-analysis of randomised controlled trials. Br J Sports Med. 2013;48:871–7.
36. Monajati A, Larumbe-Zabala E, Goss-Sampson M, Naclerio F. The effectiveness of injury prevention programs to modify risk factors for non-contact anterior cruciate ligament and hamstring injuries in uninjured team sports athletes: a systematic review. PLoS One. 2016; https://doi.org/10.1371/journal.pone.0155272.
37. Page P. Current concepts in muscle stretching for exercise and rehabilitation. Int J Sports Phys Ther. 2012;7(1):109–19.
38. Behm DG, Blazevich AJ, Kay AD, McHugh M. Acute effects of muscle stretching on physical performance, range of motion, and injury incidence in healthy active individuals: a systematic review. Appl Physiol Nutr Metab. 2016;41:1–11.
39. Chaabene H, Behm DG, Negra Y, Granacher U. Acute effects of static stretching on muscle strength and power: an attempt to clarify previous caveats. Front Physiol. 2019; https://doi.org/10.3389/fphys.2019.01468.
40. O'Sullivan K, Murray E, Sainsbury D. The effect of warm-up, static stretching and dynamic stretching on hamstring flexibility in previously injured subjects. BMC Musculoskelet Disord. 2009; https://doi.org/10.1186/1471-2474-10-37.
41. Hindle K, Whitcomb T, Briggs W, Hong J. Proprioceptive neuromuscular facilitation (PNF): its mechanisms and effects on range of motion and muscular function. J Hum Kinet. 2012;31:105–13.
42. Arnason A, Andersen TE, Holme I, Engebretsen L, Bahr R. Prevention of hamstring strains in elite soccer: an intervention study. Scand J Med Sci Sports. 2007;18:40–8.

43. Bourne MN, Timmins RG, Opar DA, Pizzari T, Ruddy JD, Sims C, Williams MD, Shield AJ. An evidence-based framework for strengthening exercises to prevent hamstring injury. Sports Med. 2017;48:251–67.
44. Hortobagyi T, Katch FI. Eccentric and concentric torque-velocity relationships during arm flexion and extension. Eur J Appl Physiol Occup Physiol. 1990;60:395–401.
45. Friden J, Lieber RL. Structural and mechanical basis of exercise-induced muscle injury. Med Sci Sports Exerc. 1992; https://doi.org/10.1249/00005768-199205000-00005.
46. Clarkson PM, Hubal MJ. Exercise-induced muscle damage in humans. Am J Phys Med Rehabil. 2002; https://doi.org/10.1097/00002060-200211001-00007.
47. Rosemeyer JR, Hayes BT, Switzler CL, Hicks-Little CA. Effects of core-musculature fatigue on maximal shoulder strength. J Sport Rehabil. 2015;24:384–90.
48. Black AM, Hagel BE, Palacios-Derflingher L, Schneider KJ, Emery CA. The risk of injury associated with body checking among Pee Wee ice hockey players: an evaluation of Hockey Canada's national body checking policy change. Br J Sports Med. 2017;51:1767–72.
49. World Rugby approves law trials to further injury-prevention. SA Rugby; 2019. https://www.sarugby.co.za/en/articles/2019/08/08/World-Rugby-approves-new-law-trials. Accessed 2 Feb 2021.
50. Dizon JM, Reyes JJ. A systematic review on the effectiveness of external ankle supports in the prevention of inversion ankle sprains among elite and recreational players. J Sci Med Sport. 2010;13:309–17.
51. Russell K, Hagel B, Francescutti LH. The effect of wrist guards on wrist and arm injuries among snowboarders: a systematic review. Clin J Sport Med. 2007;17:145–50.
52. Ekstrand J. Keeping your top players on the pitch: the key to football medicine at a professional level. Br J Sports Med. 2013;47:723–4.
53. Chakrabarti S. What's in a name? Compliance, adherence and concordance in chronic psychiatric disorders. World J Psychiatry. 2014;4:30.
54. Female esports watchers gain 6% in gender viewership share in last two years. Interpret; 2019. https://interpret.la/female-esports-watchers-gain-6-in-gender-viewership-share-in-last-two-years/. Accessed 2 Feb 2021.

Esports Cultural Competence

10

Caitlin McGee

10.1 Gaming Versus Esports Culture

A particularly important cultural distinction must be drawn between gaming and esports. This is not to suggest that the two cultures are entirely separate from one another; there are a variety of shared health and physical performance concerns. However, esports competitors face added demands in the same way that professional Women's National Basketball Association players face demands that casual players in a game of pickup basketball do not. These demands are related to the increased quality and frequency of play as well as ancillary concerns resulting from full-time employment as an esports competitor. Players may have sponsorship or streaming obligations in addition to their scheduled practices, must deal with the stresses of travel for tournaments, and grapple with the psychological impact of competition.

In previous chapters of this textbook, the importance of knowing the specific musculoskeletal strains that players face was emphasized. This includes knowing what game title the patient plays, what peripherals (mouse, keyboard, controller, etc.) they use, how often they practice and play, what their tournament

C. McGee (✉)
1HP, Washington, DC, USA

© The Author(s), under exclusive license to Springer Nature
Switzerland AG 2021
L. Migliore et al. (eds.), *Handbook of Esports Medicine*,
https://doi.org/10.1007/978-3-030-73610-1_10

241

schedule is, and what other non-gaming activities they do on a daily basis that might load the same tissues. However, the musculoskeletal component is not the only component of load or strain. An intervention that is concerned solely with the physiological impact of gaming falls short of addressing players' needs. Without a robust understanding of and respect for the full picture of what loads esports competitors carry, return to play program designs will be lacking.

Consider programming for return to sport in traditional sports athletes status post anterior cruciate ligament reconstruction (ACLR). The exact timeline and appropriate metrics for full return to sport remain a hotly debated topic in the world of sports medicine. Research indicates that players with fear of movement, fear of reinjury, and lack of confidence are correlated with lower strength scores, decreased overall activity, increased injury risk, altered movement patterns, and poorer performance when returning to play [1, 2, 3, 4]. As previously discussed, research in esports medicine and performance is lacking, and often best practices must be applied from analogous fields. In this case, it is reasonable to extrapolate the importance of addressing kinesiophobia in all competitive athletes, both traditional and esports.

In treating a patient with an ACLR, there are certain aspects of the plan of care which will be consistent across all patients. Postsurgical protocols address tissue healing times that do not vary significantly from a professional athlete to a weekend warrior. However, certain aspects of the plan of care are goal-dependent. While a casual gamer may experience frustration, fear of movement, or anxiety in response to an injury that limits their ability to play, a professional esports competitor faces additional stresses due to the risk to their career and their standing in the community or on a team. Research has demonstrated a clear link between anxiety and increased perception of pain across a variety of injury types, and current models of pain management emphasize an approach that considers not just physiological factors but also social influences, psychological factors, economic difficulties, and perceived self-efficacy [5, 6, 7, 8]. Best practice in the treatment of professional esports competitors should, therefore, factor in how esports culture shapes the attitudes and perspectives of these patients.

10.2   Professional Development

One area in which traditional sports differs significantly from esports is in development, or the "path to pro." Traditional sports have a variety of developmental avenues: club/intramural leagues, travel leagues, high school varsity programs, collegiate varsity programs, etc. It is highly likely that, even if athletes have not personally dealt with injuries, they have meaningfully interacted with or at least observed their teammates' interactions with medical professionals (e.g., athletic trainers, physical therapists, or physicians).

In stark contrast, very few developmental programs exist for esports. A few adult amateur leagues exist, but they are the functional equivalent of adult coed leagues for soccer. The largest exception to this would be the Faceit Pro League (FPL) Circuit, an independent system of in-house leagues designed to create opportunities for amateur and professional players to play together [9]. Currently, the FPL Circuit operates Dota 2, Counter-Strike: Global Offensive, and Rainbow Six Siege leagues. A small number of professional organizations have "academy" or "contenders" teams akin to AAA teams in baseball. In some titles, such as Overwatch or League of Legends, these teams compete in separate Contenders or Academy Leagues [10, 11].

While these systems offer opportunities for players to grow and develop with regards to mechanical skill, teamwork, communication, game strategy, and competitive performance, there is no specific health or injury prevention infrastructure to support them or to introduce players to out-of-game aspects of professional play.

More recently, high schools and colleges have begun to establish both club and varsity esports programs, bolstered by organizations such as the High School Esports League, Play VS, North America Scholastic Esports Federation, and the Electronic Gaming Federation. In the past 2–5 years, a small number of colleges have begun to offer scholarships for varsity esports competitors. Some collegiate teams compete exclusively in collegiate leagues; others compete in both collegiate leagues and in professional leagues. Notably, the NCAA is not involved in collegiate esports [12]. This is generally seen as a net positive by members of the esports community. It also means, however, that there is no central regulatory body developing health and performance standards for players and schools. Some collegiate programs are under the auspices of the athletics departments; others are considered the domain of student life departments. This results in significant discrepancies concerning familiarity with healthcare professionals, and subsequent care.

For many players, this lack of familiarity breeds skepticism of the necessity of healthcare professionals. This attitude is best summed up as "I got to a professional level without you, why do I need you now?" As a result, education and rapport-building are particularly key components of esports medicine.

This skepticism of non-endemic entities is not exclusive to healthcare providers and should not be seen as a skepticism of medicine as a whole. Rather, the issue is twofold: many esports competitors are skeptical of the insufficiently-prepared providers they are likely to have encountered, and the esports community as a whole is cautious of any individual or organization they perceive as an outsider. This latter component is reasonable when considering the number of organizations and tournaments which have scammed players or the number of individuals who claim to be esports experts on LinkedIn and on conference panels without any day-to-day experience in the industry [13, 14].

The former component—skepticism as a result of poor previous experiences with medical professionals—is not unfounded. Esports medicine is a remarkably new field. Even setting aside the issues of financial considerations, the complexities of insurance, and general access to care, relatively few providers have significant experience working with gaming populations, let alone esports competitors. In the authors' practice, patients have reported several experiences with ignorant providers who do not fully understand the implications of their treatment recommendations. Examples include a consistent report of having been instructed to wear a brace rather than seek therapy, to solely rest without any other recommendations, or to just stop playing games entirely. Other athletes have been informed that surgical procedures are the only solution to their pain, leaving them reluctant to seek out care for other injuries in the future.

It is not, strictly speaking, necessary for a well-qualified medical professional to have personal experience in gaming or esports, any more than it is necessary for a well-qualified sports medicine professional to have played the sports of the athletes they treat. It is unquestionably necessary that best practices in esports, as in traditional sports, involve understanding the biological, psychological, and social demands of professionals receiving treatment. Direct gaming experience can be helpful to establish a baseline of common ground and to allow the care provider to speak knowledgeably about their patient's competitive arena. Given the skepticism discussed above, such experience is also likely to promote an improved patient-provider relationship and establish a degree of credibility for the care provider.

10.3 Current Practice Routines

Professional esports competitors' practice schedules are dramatically different from those of professional traditional sports competitors. In traditional sports, no professional teams would consider practicing for 8+ hours a day, every day, or of coming home and playing a game of pickup football for fun after a day of practicing. This is not only common in esports, it is widely accepted by players as the most effective practice model for success.

Professional gamers across a variety of teams and titles describe schedules that involve 5–8 hours per day of team practice, 1–2 hours of video review and game strategy discussion, and 2–3 hours of solo gaming time, usually on the title they play professionally [15, 16, 17]. This model of practice has its origins in the Korean esports scene, and requires some historical context to explain.

While certainly not the only country to develop a robust esports scene, South Korea has historically been regarded as one of the most dominant competitive regions in esports [18]. This was, in part, because of the extent to which competitive game titles like StarCraft: Brood War were not only adopted by teens and young adults but also broadcasted by mainstream television sources [19].

Across a variety of game titles, from StarCraft to League of Legends, South Korean players and teams consistently dominated.

As non-Korean players looked to make their own mark in esports, they adopted many of the same practices as their South Korean counterparts, including their practice schedules. Per the coach of Gen.G Esports, one of South Korea's premier esports organizations, players train 12 to 15 hours per day in season and at least 8 hours per day in the off-season [17]. This schedule is not an outlier in the Korean model of esports practice; it is considered the norm.

While some teams have begun to move away from such a demanding schedule, there is still significant buy-in to this model from professional and aspiring esports competitors. It has demonstrably worked, for certain values of "worked" – that is to say, professionals who have followed this model have had significant competitive success in esports. Given the widespread acceptance of the efficacy of this practice structure, care providers may experience pushback to attempted modifications incorporating research on training periodization and cognitive load.

This is not to suggest that such modifications should not be made. However, as previously stated, it is imperative to understand the broader context of a player's and a team's load and decisions. In this case, knowledge of the reasons for these schedules allows for a more nuanced and less abrupt approach to change, which is likely to result in a better outcome.

10.4   Caveat

As is likely clear in this chapter, the esports community has a unique culture with in-group beliefs, biases, and memes. While a general overview is possible, in-depth understanding requires participation. It is possible to provide adequate care for musculoskeletal injuries based solely on orthopedic principles and a knowledge of the biomechanical forces which shape physiological load in esports competitors. However, with or without in-depth understanding of the community, medical professionals must respect the broader social and cultural forces endemic to esports that shape the perspectives of their patients if they intend to provide effective, meaningful, patient-centered care.

References

1. Hart HF, Culvenor AG, Guermazi A, Crossley KM. Worse knee confidence, fear of movement, psychological readiness to return-to-sport and pain are associated with worse function after ACL reconstruction. Phys Ther Sport. 2020;41:1–8. https://doi.org/10.1016/j.ptsp.2019.10.006.
2. Paterno MV, Flynn K, Thomas S, Schmitt LC. Self-reported fear predicts functional performance and second ACL injury after ACL reconstruction and return to sport: a pilot study. Sports Health. 2018;10(3):228–33. https://doi.org/10.1177/1941738117745806.
3. Lentz TA, Zeppieri G Jr, George SZ, Tillman SM, Moser MW, Farmer KW, et al. Comparison of physical impairment, functional, and psychosocial measures based on fear of reinjury/lack of confidence and return-to-sport status after ACL reconstruction. Am J Sports Med. 2015;43(2):345–53. https://doi.org/10.1177/0363546514559707.
4. Zarzycki R, Failla M, Capin J, Snyder-Mackle L. Psychological readiness to return to sport is associated with knee kinematic asymmetry during gait following ACL reconstruction. J Orthop Sports Phys Ther. 2018;48:1–21. https://doi.org/10.2519/jospt.2018.8084.
5. Bevers K, Watts L, Kishino N, Gatchel R. The biopsychosocial model of the assessment, prevention, and treatment of chronic pain. US Neurol. 2016;12:98. https://doi.org/10.17925/USN.2016.12.02.98.
6. Gorczyca R, Filip R, Walczak E. Psychological aspects of pain. Ann Agric Environ Med. 2013;(Spec no. 1):23–7.
7. Bletzer J, Gantz S, Voigt T, Neubauer E, Schiltenwolf M. Chronische untere Rückenschmerzen und psychische Komorbidität: Eine Übersicht [Chronic low back pain and psychological comorbidity: a review]. Schmerz. 2017;31(2):93–101. German. https://doi.org/10.1007/s00482-016-0143-4. PMID: 27501800.
8. Thibodeau MA, Welch PG, Katz J, Asmundson GJG. Pain-related anxiety influences pain perception differently in men and women: a quantitative sensory test across thermal pain modalities. Pain. 2013;154(3):419–26. https://doi.org/10.1016/j.pain.2012.12.001.
9. FPL Circuit. 2018. https://pro.faceit.com. Accessed 22 Feb 2021.
10. Overwatch Contenders. 2020. https://overwatchleague.com/en-us/contenders. Accessed 22 Feb 2021.
11. LCS Academy League. 2021. https://liquipedia.net/leagueoflegends/LCS/Academy_League. Accessed 22 Feb 2021.

12. Hayward A. NCAA votes to not govern collegiate esports. 2019. https://esportsobserver.com/ncaa-nogo-collegiate-esports. Accessed 22 Feb 2021.

13. Byers P. 2019. Denial Esports allegedly owes over €100,000 in salaries and for CWL Pro League payment. https://dotesports.com/call-of-duty/news/denial-esports-owes-salaries-pro-league. Accessed 22 Feb 2021.

14. Competitive ruling: renegades and TDK. 2015. https://nexus.leagueoflegends.com/en-us/2016/05/competitive-ruling-renegades-and-tdk. Accessed 22 Feb 2021.

15. Intel. The daily regimen of players in professional gaming. 2017. https://www.intel.com/content/www/us/en/gaming/resources/gamer-life.html. Accessed 22 Feb 2021.

16. Jacobs H. Here's the insane training schedule of a 20-something professional gamer. 2015. https://www.businessinsider.com/pro-gamers-explain-the-insane-training-regimen-they-use-to-stay-on-top-2015-5. Accessed 22 Feb 2021.

17. Lambrechts S. Pro gamers in South Korea train for 15 hours a day – here's what's involved. 2019. https://www.techradar.com/news/pro-gamers-in-south-korea-train-for-15-hours-a-day-heres-whats-involved. Accessed 22 Feb 2021.

18. Barretts B. League of Legends Worlds 2016 finals are Korea vs. Korea once again as SKT look to form a dynasty. 2016. https://www.pcgamesn.com/league-of-legends/league-of-legends-worlds-2016-finals-skt-samsung. Accessed 22 Feb 2021.

19. Leandre K. How Korea embraced eSports and haven't looked back. 2015. https://sea.ign.com/esports/92089/feature/how-korea-embraced-esports-and-havent-looked-back. Accessed 22 Feb 2021.

Index

A
Action real-time strategy (ARTS), 11
Addiction, 191–193
Aggression, 190

B
Biodynamics, 224
Biomechanics, 224–226

C
Carpometacarpal (CMC), 49
Common peroneal nerve, 143
Compressive neuropathies, 142
Computer gaming, 7
Console controller, 158, 159
Console gaming, 5

D
Daily fueling, 172, 174, 175
Deep vein thrombosis, 125, 126, 128, 132
Digital collectible card games (DCCGs), 12
Digital games, 187–189
    aggression, 190
    cognitive impact, 189
    psychological well-being, 190, 195
    skill development, 195
    violent crime, 191, 193, 194
Dynamic stretching, 230